# A Fitness Nutrition Book

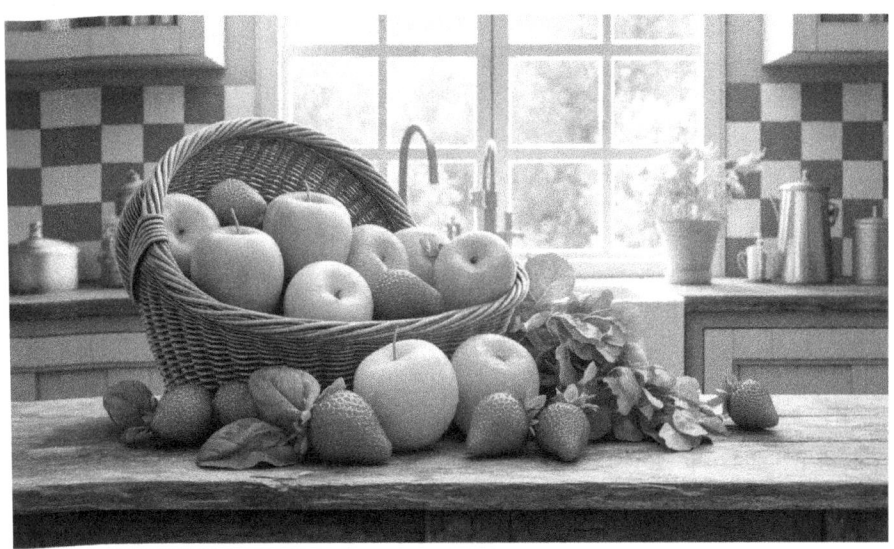

CRAFTED BY SKRIUWER

**Copyright © 2025 by Skriuwer.**

All rights reserved. No part of this book may be used or reproduced in any form whatsoever without written permission except in the case of brief quotations in critical articles or reviews.

At **Skriuwer**, we're more than just a team—we're a global community of people who love books. In Frisian, "Skriuwer" means "writer," and that's at the heart of what we do: creating and sharing books with readers worldwide. Wherever you are in the world, **Skriuwer** is here to inspire learning.

**Frisian** is one of the oldest languages in Europe, closely related to English and Dutch, and is spoken by about **500,000 people** in the province of **Friesland** (Fryslân), located in the northern Netherlands. It's the second official language of the Netherlands, but like many minority languages, Frisian faces the challenge of survival in a modern, globalized world.

We're using the money we earn to promote the Frisian language.

For more information, contact : **kontakt@skriuwer.com** (www.skriuwer.com)

# TABLE OF CONTENTS

## CHAPTER 1: UNDERSTANDING FOOD AND YOUR BODY

- Essential nutrients and their roles
- How digestion works and why it matters
- Overview of main food groups

## CHAPTER 2: BASICS OF HEALTHFUL EATING

- Forming balanced meals
- Portion control strategies
- Building simpler, healthier habits

## CHAPTER 3: PROTEINS: BUILDING BLOCKS FOR STRONG MUSCLES

- Why proteins are crucial
- Animal vs. plant protein sources
- Signs and impact of low protein

## CHAPTER 4: CARBOHYDRATES: FUEL FOR ACTIVE DAYS

- Differences between complex and simple carbs
- Importance of whole grains and fiber
- Balancing carb intake for energy

## CHAPTER 5: FATS: IMPORTANCE OF HEALTHY SOURCES

- Unsaturated, saturated, and trans fats explained
- Healthier cooking methods
- Ways to include good fats in meals

## CHAPTER 6: VITAMINS: TINY HELPERS FOR BIG NEEDS

- *Fat-soluble vs. water-soluble vitamins*
- *Primary vitamins and their functions*
- *Tips to avoid vitamin deficiencies*

---

## CHAPTER 7: MINERALS: KEY TO SUPPORTING YOUR BODY

- *Major vs. trace minerals*
- *Roles of iron, calcium, potassium, and more*
- *Foods and habits for mineral balance*

---

## CHAPTER 8: WATER: WHY STAYING HYDRATED MATTERS

- *Critical role of water in the body*
- *Recognizing signs of dehydration*
- *Strategies for balanced fluid intake*

---

## CHAPTER 9: CREATING BALANCED MEALS

- *Simple plate division method*
- *Combining proteins, carbs, and fats*
- *Meal planning tips and batch cooking*

---

## CHAPTER 10: EATING WELL ON A BUDGET

- *Money-saving meal strategies*
- *Smart shopping and planning*
- *Reducing food waste to stretch resources*

## CHAPTER 11: PLANNING YOUR DAILY FOOD ROUTINE

- *Why regular meal times help*
- *Identifying true hunger vs. fullness*
- *Adapting schedules for busy lifestyles*

## CHAPTER 12: SMART SNACKING AND SWEET TREATS

- *Purpose of snacks and moderation*
- *Ideas for healthier snack options*
- *Handling sweet cravings responsibly*

## CHAPTER 13: MUSCLE GAIN THROUGH HEALTHY EATING

- *Protein's role in muscle building*
- *Balancing calories for muscle vs. fat*
- *Vegetarian and vegan muscle tips*

## CHAPTER 14: SUPPORTING WEIGHT CONTROL

- *Importance of calorie balance*
- *Gradual, steady weight changes*
- *Lifestyle strategies over quick fixes*

## CHAPTER 15: BUILDING A STRONG HEART AND BODY

- *Heart-friendly nutrients and fats*
- *Managing sodium for blood pressure*
- *Daily habits that strengthen heart health*

## CHAPTER 16: KEEPING ENERGY LEVELS STEADY

- *Preventing energy spikes and crashes*
- *Combining macros with hydration*
- *Sleep and stress influence on energy*

## CHAPTER 17: EATING TO FEEL GOOD INSIDE AND OUT

- *How food affects mood and outlook*
- *Supporting skin, hair, and gut health*
- *Boosting confidence with balanced habits*

## CHAPTER 18: MANAGING FOOD CHOICES IN DAILY LIFE

- *Meal prep and grocery planning*
- *Strategies for restaurants and gatherings*
- *Adapting to special diets and busy schedules*

## CHAPTER 19: NUTRITIONAL TIPS FOR ALL AGES

- *Unique needs for kids and teens*
- *Midlife considerations and changing demands*
- *Focus on nutrition for older adults*

## CHAPTER 20: PUTTING IT ALL TOGETHER

- *Recap of core principles*
- *Staying motivated over time*
- *Practical steps for long-term success*

# CHAPTER 1

## Understanding Food and Your Body

Food is the fuel that keeps your body moving and strong. When you eat something, it becomes part of your body's energy supply. This energy helps you walk, play, run, and do everything you enjoy. Food is also important for growth, repair, and keeping all your body parts working as they should. It is not only about filling your stomach, but also about giving your body what it needs to stay healthy.

### Why Our Bodies Need Food

Think of your body like a machine. Machines need power to run. A car needs gas to move, and your body needs energy from the foods you eat. When you eat, your body breaks down the foods into smaller pieces that enter your blood. These small pieces give power to your muscles, your brain, and other organs.

Food is more than energy alone. Certain parts of food help build muscles and other tissues. Some parts help protect you from feeling sick. Other parts keep your brain sharp, so you can remember things and learn new stuff. Many foods also help you feel satisfied, so you have enough strength to do your daily tasks.

### What Are Nutrients?

Foods contain different things called nutrients. Nutrients are important for health and growth. Here are the main groups of nutrients:

1. **Proteins:** They help build and fix muscles, skin, and other tissues.

2. **Carbohydrates:** They are the main source of energy for your body.

3. **Fats:** They give your body another source of energy. They also help your body absorb some vitamins.

4. **Vitamins:** They support many different body functions, like seeing in the dark and healing wounds.

5. **Minerals:** They help your body in many ways, such as keeping your bones strong or helping your nerves work.

6. **Water:** It is not always counted as a nutrient in the same way as the others, but it is vital. Water helps carry nutrients around your body and helps remove waste.

Your body does not treat all foods the same way. That is why choosing the right types of foods is important. If you eat too many foods that have little nutrition, your body may not get what it needs. If you eat a variety of foods with good nutrients, your body has a better chance to stay strong and healthy.

## The Role of Energy in the Body

Energy from food is measured in something called calories. A calorie is a unit that shows how much energy is in a certain food. When you do activities like running, climbing, or even thinking, you use calories. The more you move, the more calories you need. If you do not move a lot, you do not need as many calories.

But remember, calories alone do not tell you if a food is good for you. A piece of cake might have many calories, but it may not have as many vitamins or minerals compared to a bowl of mixed vegetables. Your body needs both energy and helpful nutrients. Choosing foods that have good nutrients helps your body in the long run.

## Basic Body Parts and How Food Helps Them

Your body has many parts that depend on what you eat. Here are a few important parts:

1. **Bones:** Bones need minerals like calcium and phosphorus. You often get them from foods like milk, yogurt, cheese, or leafy greens. These minerals help keep bones hard and strong.

2. **Muscles:** Muscles get help from protein, which comes from foods such as beans, eggs, fish, or lean meats. Protein helps muscles repair themselves after exercise.

3. **Brain:** The brain uses carbohydrates for energy. It also needs healthy fats and certain vitamins. Foods like whole grains, nuts, and fruits give your brain long-lasting energy.

4. **Heart:** The heart is a muscle. It needs nutrients like potassium, found in bananas or potatoes, and healthy fats from nuts or avocados to keep it working well.

5. **Skin:** Vitamins A and C help keep skin in good shape. You find these in carrots, oranges, and many other colorful fruits and vegetables.

By giving your body enough of each type of nutrient, you help support every part, from your hair down to your toes.

## How the Body Uses Food: Digestion and Absorption

When you chew and swallow, food goes into your stomach. There, acids and other substances break it down. After the stomach, the food moves to the small intestine. This is where nutrients get absorbed into your blood. Then, your blood carries these nutrients to every cell in your body.

This process is called digestion. It is like taking a big piece of something and breaking it into small pieces that your body can use. If you eat foods with lots of helpful nutrients, your cells get better supplies. That is why it is not just about eating enough food, but eating the right types of food.

## Different Food Groups

People often talk about the main food groups. While details can differ between countries, many experts mention the following groups:

1. **Fruits:** These include apples, bananas, berries, oranges, and more. Fruits often have vitamins like vitamin C and fiber that helps with digestion.

2. **Vegetables:** You have many choices, like spinach, carrots, broccoli, peppers, and peas. Vegetables give you vitamins, minerals, and fiber.

3. **Grains:** These are foods like bread, rice, oatmeal, and pasta. Whole grains are best because they have more fiber and nutrients.

4. **Protein Foods:** This group includes beans, eggs, fish, poultry, and lean meats. It also includes nuts and seeds.

5. **Dairy or Dairy Alternatives:** Milk, cheese, and yogurt are common dairy foods. If you do not eat dairy, there are dairy-free alternatives like soy milk or almond milk that may have similar nutrients.

These groups are a simple way to remember different types of foods. Choosing a mix from each group can help your body get what it needs.

## Natural Foods vs. Highly Processed Foods

You may hear people talking about natural foods. These are foods that are closer to their original state. For example, an apple is a natural food. Apple pie might still have some of the apple, but it has added sugar and other ingredients. Potato chips are even more processed. They start as potatoes but go through many steps that change their nutrient content.

Natural foods usually have more vitamins, minerals, and fiber compared to highly processed snacks. Processed foods often have extra salt, sugar, or fats that do not help your body much. You do not have to avoid these foods entirely, but you should not have them too often. Most of your meals should include foods that give you good nutrients.

## Why Food Choices Matter for Growth and Health

Children and teens need to grow. Adults need to maintain a healthy body. Older folks need to stay strong in their later years. Each group may have different needs, but everybody does best when they eat well. If you do not get enough of certain nutrients, you might feel tired or weak. If you eat too much of some things, you might have problems like extra weight or heart issues. A balance is best.

For example, if you eat a lot of sugary snacks and drinks, you might get energy spikes. You feel excited and awake for a short time. Then, you can feel tired or restless when the sugar rush wears off. If you have a balanced snack, like fruit with peanut butter or cheese and whole-grain crackers, you get longer-lasting energy without a big crash later.

## Understanding Food Labels

Many foods in stores have labels that show you how much protein, carbohydrates, fats, vitamins, and minerals are in each serving. These labels also show you how many calories each serving has. Learning to read these labels can help you choose foods that fit your needs. You can compare two similar products to see which one has less sugar or more fiber. We will talk more about selecting healthy foods in later chapters, but know that these labels can be helpful.

## How Food Affects Your Mood and Mind

Have you ever felt grouchy when you skipped a meal? Or maybe you felt too full and sleepy after eating a big meal? That is because food can affect how you feel. When you do not eat enough or when you eat foods with too much sugar, your mood can go up and down quickly. Eating well can help you feel more stable and happy. Having enough protein, healthy fats, vitamins, and minerals makes a difference not just in your body, but also in your mind.

## Activity Levels and Food Choices

If you like to play sports or run around the yard, your body might need more energy. If you mostly read books or watch shows, you might not need as many calories in a day. Pay attention to your daily activities. If you do more active things, you need more calories and protein. If you are less active, watch your portion sizes. Eating more than you burn can lead to extra weight. Your body does store energy as fat, which is normal, but too much stored fat can put strain on your heart and other organs over time.

## Important Tips for a Balanced Start

1. **Eat a variety of foods:** Try different fruits, vegetables, grains, and protein sources. Different foods have different nutrients.

2. **Listen to your body:** Eat when you are hungry and stop when you are satisfied, not overly stuffed.

3. **Stay hydrated:** Water is key for digestion, carrying nutrients, and keeping your body temperature steady.

4. **Be mindful of treats:** Sugary or salty snacks are okay sometimes, but they should not take the place of healthier choices.

## Common Myths About Food

1. **Myth:** If a food package says "low fat," it means the food is healthy.
   **Truth:** Some low-fat foods have extra sugar or salt to make them taste better. Always check the nutrient facts.

2. **Myth:** Skipping meals helps you manage your weight.
   **Truth:** Missing meals can make you overeat later or choose less healthy snacks. It is usually better to have regular meals with balanced nutrients.

3. **Myth:** Protein bars or shakes are necessary for everyone who wants to be healthy.
   **Truth:** While these can help some people, many folks can get enough protein from regular meals that include beans, eggs, fish, and lean meats.

## Being Kind to Your Body

Eating well means you are being kind to your body. You show kindness by giving it foods that help you move, think, and play. If you fill up on junk food, your body might not work as smoothly as it could. By focusing on a mix of healthy foods, you can keep feeling good and stay active. This does not mean you can never have a cookie or a slice of pizza. It just means you keep those choices in moderation.

## The Social Side of Eating

Eating is also a social activity. Families and friends share meals and talk about their day. Different cultures have special foods for festivals and celebrations. Learning about foods from different places can be fun and help you find new things to taste. Trying different dishes that include vegetables, grains, or healthy proteins can open your eyes to new flavors and textures.

## What Happens If You Do Not Get Enough Nutrients?

If you do not eat enough protein, your muscles and tissues might not fix themselves as easily. If you skip out on key vitamins and minerals, you might get tired more often or get sick more easily. Your body needs certain nutrients to keep your heart healthy, your bones strong, and your brain working well. That is why balanced meals are important.

## Signs of Poor Eating Habits

- **Feeling Tired:** If you lack vitamins or eat too many sugary foods, you might feel tired all the time.
- **Frequent Illnesses:** Your immune system needs nutrients to fight off germs.

- **Mood Changes:** Foods that are too high in sugar or missing important nutrients can cause sudden mood swings.

- **Weight Problems:** Eating too much junk food or not having enough nutritious meals can lead to weight gain or weight loss that is not healthy.

## Eating Patterns that Support Your Body

Since your body needs consistent energy, many people choose to eat a few meals a day along with small snacks if needed. You do not have to eat the same number of meals as everyone else, but spacing out your meals helps your body use the energy and nutrients properly. If you wait too long between meals, you might get too hungry and eat too fast, which can upset your stomach.

## The Joy of Knowing What Your Body Needs

Learning about your body and how food helps it can be exciting. You start to notice that when you eat better, you feel better. You might see that your hair feels stronger, your nails are not as brittle, and your skin looks brighter. Inside your body, your heart and brain also do better with the right nutrients. Even though you cannot see these parts directly, they depend on what you choose to eat.

## Putting It All Together

Your body is like a wonderful system, ready to keep you active, help you learn, and give you the strength to face each day. But it can only do this well if it gets the right fuel. Understanding the basics of food and your body is the first step to making better choices that will help you in many areas of your life. You do not have to give up everything you love to eat. You just need to pay attention to what your body needs. In the chapters ahead, we will learn more about how different nutrients work and how to make balanced choices.

# CHAPTER 2

## Basics of Healthful Eating

Eating well can feel confusing if you are not sure where to start. But it does not have to be hard. Healthful eating means choosing foods that help your body in the best ways possible. It also means enjoying what you eat. You can keep your meals simple and still get all the good things you need.

## What Does "Healthful" Mean?

When people say "healthful food," they often mean foods that are natural, not full of extra sugar or salt, and have a good balance of nutrients. It does not mean you can only eat vegetables and never have a treat. It is about making sure that the main part of your daily diet supports your body. You can still enjoy special snacks or desserts sometimes, but they should not be your main source of calories.

## Building Balanced Meals

A balanced meal has a mix of foods that give you protein, carbohydrates, fats, vitamins, and minerals. One easy way to imagine a balanced meal is to look at your plate. Think about dividing it into sections:

- Half of your plate for colorful vegetables and fruits.

- About one-quarter of your plate for protein foods.

- About one-quarter of your plate for whole grains or starchy vegetables like potatoes.

This is not a strict rule for every single meal. But it helps you remember to add some veggies or fruits, include a source of protein, and pick a healthy grain. You can adjust the amounts based on what your body needs.

## Simple Ways to Include More Fruits and Vegetables

1. **Add fruit to your breakfast:** Sliced bananas, strawberries, or apples go well with cereal or oatmeal.

2. **Snack on cut-up veggies:** Carrot sticks, cucumber slices, or bell pepper strips make an easy snack.

3. **Mix veggies into your main meals:** You can add spinach or peas to pasta. You can top your pizza with mushrooms or peppers.

4. **Try different colors:** Each color of vegetable or fruit can offer different nutrients. Red, green, orange, yellow, and purple foods all have unique benefits.

## Understanding Whole Grains

Whole grains keep all parts of the grain kernel. This means they have more fiber, vitamins, and minerals than refined grains. Good examples of whole grains include:

- Whole wheat bread

- Oatmeal

- Brown rice

- Quinoa

Refined grains, like white bread or white rice, go through a process that takes away some parts of the grain. These refined products might still have some nutrients, but they lose fiber and other important parts. Fiber helps you feel full and helps keep your digestion regular. That is why choosing more whole grains is often better.

## Healthy Protein Choices

Protein is necessary for building and fixing your body's tissues. Some good protein choices include:

- Lean meats like chicken or turkey

- Fish and seafood

- Beans and lentils

- Tofu or tempeh

- Eggs

- Nuts and seeds

Eating a variety of these helps you get different nutrients. If you do not eat meat, you can get protein from beans, lentils, tofu, nuts, and seeds. Try to choose lean cuts of meat to reduce the amount of saturated fat.

## Importance of Healthy Fats

Some people think all fats are bad, but that is not true. Your body needs certain fats to help with energy, absorb vitamins, and keep cells healthy. The main thing is to choose the right kinds of fats:

- **Unsaturated fats:** Found in foods like avocados, nuts, seeds, and olive oil. They can be helpful for heart health.

- **Saturated fats:** Often found in butter, high-fat meats, and cheese. These should be limited because they can affect your heart if you eat too much.

- **Trans fats:** These are often in some snack foods and fried foods. They can be very harmful. Many places have reduced or removed trans fats from foods.

## Portion Sizes

Even when eating healthy foods, portion size matters. If you eat too much of anything, you might gain extra weight or feel stuffed. If you eat too little, you might not get enough nutrients. A helpful strategy is to begin with smaller amounts and only go back for more if you are still hungry.

## Eating Slowly and Enjoying Meals

When you eat fast, you might not realize you are full until you have had too much. Taking your time can help you notice when you are satisfied. Enjoy the flavors, colors, and smells of your meal. This also gives your brain time to understand that your stomach has food. When you rush, you can miss the signals that say, "Enough."

## Healthy Eating in Everyday Life

You do not have to make big, complicated meals to eat well. You can keep things easy:

- **Breakfast:** Whole-grain cereal or oatmeal with fruit and low-fat milk.

- **Lunch:** A sandwich on whole-grain bread with lean meat or beans, plus some vegetables.

- **Dinner:** Lean protein like chicken or fish, whole-grain pasta or brown rice, and steamed vegetables.

Snacks could be fruit, yogurt, or nuts. Remember to drink water regularly. This pattern makes sure you are getting a good mix of nutrients throughout the day.

## Checking Food Labels for a Better Choice

Food labels can help you see if a product has lots of added sugar, salt, or unhealthy fats. When comparing two items, pick the one with less sugar, less salt, or fewer unhealthy fats. For example, if you like yogurt, compare a sweetened fruit yogurt with a plain yogurt plus fresh fruit. The sweetened fruit yogurt may have a lot of added sugar, while plain yogurt with your own fruit often has less added sugar.

## Why Excess Sugar and Salt Can Be a Problem

Eating too much sugar can cause spikes in energy followed by crashes. Over time, it can also lead to weight gain and other health issues. Too much salt can affect blood pressure. Many processed foods have hidden salt and sugar. That is why preparing meals at home can help you control how much of these you eat.

## Planning Ahead for Healthy Choices

If you want to do well in sports, you might practice ahead of time. Eating well also benefits from planning. If you plan out your meals for the week, you are less likely to grab junk food at the last minute. Here are simple planning tips:

- **Make a shopping list:** Write down what you need for your planned meals.

- **Buy fruits and vegetables in season:** They are often cheaper and taste better.

- **Cook in batches:** You can make a big pot of soup or stew and freeze some for later.

- **Keep healthy snacks ready:** Wash and cut fruits or vegetables in advance, so they are easy to grab.

## Eating on Special Occasions

Birthday parties, holidays, or other celebrations often have cakes, candies, or snacks. It is okay to enjoy these, but do not let them become an everyday habit. You can have a slice of cake or a cookie and still maintain healthful eating habits if you are balanced in your normal meals. The key is that these items are treats, not the main event of your daily diet.

## Eating Outside the Home

Sometimes, you might eat at restaurants or buy food while you are out. Restaurant meals can be large and may have extra butter, oils, or sauces. If you can, look for menu items that are grilled instead of fried. You can also ask for sauces on the side or skip sugary drinks. If the portion is too big, take half home for another meal. Having a rough idea of what is in your meal helps you maintain good habits.

## Learning to Enjoy Healthful Foods

Some people say they do not like vegetables, but maybe they just have not tried them in a way they enjoy. You can roast vegetables with a little oil and herbs to bring out sweet flavors. You can blend spinach into a fruit smoothie, and you might hardly taste it. Trying new methods of cooking can be fun, and you might find new favorites.

## Tips to Make Healthful Eating Tasty

1. **Add herbs and spices:** They can give flavor without adding salt or sugar.

2. **Try different cooking methods:** Baking, roasting, steaming, or grilling can change the taste and texture of foods.

3. **Combine healthy ingredients:** Put fruit in yogurt or vegetables in a soup. You can discover many fun tastes.

4. **Explore different cultures' foods:** Foods from around the world often use a wide range of ingredients, including vegetables, grains, and beans.

## How Eating Well Supports Your Goals

If you want to do better in sports, music, or even school, having the right nutrients helps you. Protein repairs muscles, healthy carbs give you energy, and vitamins support your overall health. Not eating enough or eating mostly junk food can leave you feeling slow. You may also have trouble focusing or feel tired during important tasks. By making a simple plan to eat healthier, you might see improvements in how you perform and how you feel each day.

## Staying Hydrated

Water helps every cell in your body. It carries nutrients to cells and helps carry waste away. It also helps you keep a steady body temperature. Thirst is often the first sign that your body needs water, but you do not want to wait until you are very thirsty. Drink water throughout the day, especially if you are active or if the weather is hot. While fruit juices and milk can also give you fluids, they have calories. Water has no calories, so it is often the best choice. Soda and other sweet drinks can be high in sugar, so have them sparingly.

## Common Obstacles to Healthful Eating and How to Handle Them

1. **Busy Schedules:** If you are always on the go, it can be hard to cook meals at home. Try quick meal ideas like sandwiches or wraps with lean proteins and lots of vegetables. You can also prepare a dish on the weekend and divide it into portions for the week.

2. **Cost:** Some people think eating well is expensive. But whole grains, beans, and seasonal vegetables can be affordable. Buying in bulk and cooking at home can save money.

3. **Picky Eating:** If you do not like certain foods, try to find new ways to prepare them or mix them with other flavors. You can also look for other foods in the same food group.

4. **Cravings for Junk Food:** If you are used to eating sugary or salty snacks, it can be tough to switch. Start by slowly replacing them with healthier snacks. Over time, you might find you do not miss the junk food as much.

## Learning to Listen to Your Body's Signals

Your body gives you signs about hunger and fullness. Learning to recognize these signs is key to healthful eating. If you eat only because you are bored or upset, you may take in extra calories that your body does not need. If you force yourself to keep eating when you are already full, you might feel uncomfortable. Paying attention to your hunger and fullness signals can help you avoid overeating or under-eating.

## Keeping a Food Journal (Optional)

Some people find it helpful to keep track of what they eat. You do not have to count every calorie, but writing down your meals and snacks can show you patterns. You might notice that you skip breakfast or that you eat too many sugary foods in the afternoon. Once you see your habits, you can make small changes. But not everyone enjoys writing down their meals, so it is an optional step.

## The Power of Small Changes

You do not have to change everything at once. Start by adding one more serving of fruits or vegetables each day. Switch from white bread to whole-grain bread. Drink water instead of a sugary drink once in a while. These small steps can add up over time and help you feel better. Then, you can move on to bigger changes if you want to.

## Bringing It All Together

Healthful eating is all about balance. You need enough protein to keep your muscles in good shape, whole grains and fruits for lasting energy, and plenty of vegetables for vitamins and minerals. Healthy fats also have a place in your meals. Enjoy your food, chew slowly, and pay attention to how you feel. With simple steps and a bit of planning, you can set yourself on a path that keeps you strong, active, and ready for anything that comes your way. And remember, you can still have favorite treats sometimes, as long as you build your day around foods that serve your body well.

# CHAPTER 3

## Proteins: Building Blocks for Strong Muscles

Proteins are often called the building blocks of the body. They help fix and build tissues, muscles, organs, and even hair and nails. When you exercise, do sports, or play around, your muscles can become strained. Proteins help your muscles recover and become stronger. But muscles are just one part of the story. Proteins also support hormones, enzymes, and important body processes that keep you healthy.

## What Are Proteins Exactly?

Proteins are made up of small units called amino acids. Imagine amino acids like letters of an alphabet, and a complete protein is like a word formed by putting these letters together. Your body needs a certain set of amino acids to perform its tasks. Some amino acids your body can make on its own, but others must come from food.

The amino acids you get from food help build new proteins inside your body. These proteins keep your muscles, bones, and organs in top shape. They also help your immune system fight off illnesses. If you do not get enough protein, you might feel weak or take longer to recover from exercise or injuries.

## Why Protein Matters for Everyone

1. **Muscle Repair:** After activities like running, climbing, or any sport, your muscle fibers might have small tears. Protein is needed to fix those tears and strengthen your muscles.

2. **Growth:** Children and teenagers need more protein compared to some adults because they are still growing. Proper protein intake helps them get taller and stronger.

3. **Immune System Support:** Proteins make antibodies, which help protect your body from germs. Without enough protein, you might get sick more easily.

4. **Energy (When Needed):** Carbohydrates and fats are usually the main fuel for your body. But if you do not eat enough of these, your body can break down protein for energy, which is not ideal since you need protein for other tasks.

## Complete vs. Incomplete Proteins

- **Complete Proteins:** These contain all the amino acids your body cannot make by itself. Foods like meat, fish, eggs, and dairy are complete proteins. Some plant-based foods like soy products (tofu or edamame) also count as complete.

- **Incomplete Proteins:** These are missing some of the amino acids your body needs. Beans, nuts, seeds, and many grains are incomplete on their own. But you can pair incomplete proteins to make a complete protein in your meals. For example, rice and beans together can supply all the essential amino acids.

## Animal-Based Protein Sources

1. **Lean Meats (Chicken, Turkey):** These have high protein and are lower in fat compared to some other meats. They also have iron, which helps your blood carry oxygen.

2. **Fish (Salmon, Tuna):** Fish offers protein and healthy fats that your body uses for many functions.

3. **Eggs:** One egg has a good amount of protein and important vitamins. The yolk has vitamins and minerals, while the white has most of the protein.

4. **Dairy (Milk, Cheese, Yogurt):** Dairy can be high in protein. For those who do not have dairy, there are options like fortified soy or almond milk that have added protein.

## Plant-Based Protein Sources

1. **Beans and Lentils:** Black beans, kidney beans, lentils, and chickpeas have protein and fiber. They can be used in soups, salads, or main dishes.

2. **Tofu and Tempeh:** Made from soybeans, they are complete proteins. They can take on many flavors, which makes them useful in lots of meals.

3. **Nuts and Seeds (Almonds, Pumpkin Seeds):** They have protein and healthy fats. They can be sprinkled on salads, oatmeal, or eaten as a snack.

4. **Quinoa:** A seed that people often treat like a grain. Quinoa is considered a complete protein because it has all the amino acids your body needs.

## How Much Protein Do You Need?

The amount of protein you need can vary based on your age, size, and how active you are. Kids and teens usually need more protein for growth. Adults who do heavy workouts might also need more than someone who does not exercise much. As a rough guide, many people aim to have some protein with each meal. You might see figures like 10-35% of your total calories from protein, but exact amounts depend on personal factors.

## Protein Timing

Some people wonder if it is important to have protein at a certain time of day, like right after exercise. While the total amount of protein you eat per day is most important, having some protein soon after physical activity may help fix and build muscles. You do not need to worry too much if you have balanced meals. The key is to spread your protein intake throughout the day. That way your body always has amino acids available to support its activities.

## Signs You Might Not Be Getting Enough Protein

1. **Weak Muscles or Slow Recovery:** If you feel you are not building strength or if your muscles stay sore for too long after activity.

2. **Hair and Nail Problems:** Hair and nails are made of certain proteins. If they become weak or brittle, it might be a signal.

3. **Frequent Illnesses:** If you get sick often, it could be that your immune system is not getting enough protein to make antibodies.

4. **Feeling Tired All the Time:** Protein supports many body systems. Low protein levels can affect energy and mood.

## Balancing Protein with Other Nutrients

Even though protein is important, you still need carbohydrates, healthy fats, vitamins, and minerals. If you eat only protein and ignore the other nutrients, your body will not get the full range of fuel and support it needs. A balanced meal often has a protein source, some vegetables or fruits, and a source of carbohydrates. You can add healthy fats like avocado slices or a drizzle of olive oil.

## Proteins for Special Diets

Some people choose a vegetarian or vegan diet. Others might have allergies or intolerances. If you do not eat meat, you can rely on beans, lentils, nuts, seeds, tofu, tempeh, and other plant-based proteins. It is possible to get enough protein through plants if you combine foods thoughtfully. For example, brown rice and beans together supply a good range of amino acids. You can also explore whole-grain breads with peanut butter or seeds to get protein.

## Protein and Exercise

If you play sports or enjoy running around outside, your muscles need to fix and grow. Protein is essential for helping your muscles do that. Many athletes focus on getting enough protein so they do not lose muscle. But remember, more is not always better. If you eat too much protein, your body may not use it all, and it could turn into stored energy. Extra protein can also be hard on your kidneys over a very long time. That is why balance is key.

## Easy Ways to Add More Protein to Meals

1. **Add beans to soups or salads:** A simple step that boosts the protein content.

2. **Choose Greek yogurt instead of regular yogurt:** Greek yogurt usually has more protein.

3. **Use nuts or seeds as toppings:** Sprinkle them on oatmeal, cereals, or salads.

4. **Try a serving of fish or lean meat with dinner:** Pair it with vegetables and a whole grain for a balanced plate.

5. **Consider eggs for breakfast:** An egg or two can give you a good start to the day.

## Shopping Tips for Protein Foods

- **Read labels for deli meats or processed meats:** Some have extra salt or preservatives.

- **Look for lean cuts:** If you buy red meat, try to pick leaner options with less visible fat.

- **Buy in bulk and freeze:** You can save money by purchasing larger amounts of meats or beans, then freezing or storing them in smaller portions.

- **Try new plant proteins:** If you have never had lentils or chickpeas, add them to your menu. They can be cheaper and healthier than some meats.

## Cooking Methods that Keep Protein Foods Healthy

- **Grilling or Baking:** Helps reduce extra fat, especially compared to frying.

- **Steaming or Boiling:** Good for fish or small pieces of meat, keeps them moist without extra oil.

- **Stir-Frying:** Lets you cook thin slices of meat or tofu quickly with lots of vegetables.

- **Slow Cooking:** Useful for beans, lentils, and tougher cuts of meat. It makes them tender and flavorful.

## Protein Supplements and Bars

You might see protein powders and bars in stores. They can help some people who need more protein quickly, such as athletes or those who struggle to eat enough during meals. But many people can get enough protein from their regular meals if they plan well. Protein supplements may have added sugars or artificial ingredients. If you are thinking of using them, it is best to check with a health professional or an adult who can guide you. Natural food sources often provide a wider range of nutrients than a single product.

## Protein Myths

1. **Myth:** "You have to eat loads of meat to build muscle."
   **Truth:** You do need enough protein, but balance matters more. Muscle growth also depends on exercise, not just protein intake.

2. **Myth:** "Vegetarian or vegan diets cannot give you enough protein."
   **Truth:** You can get enough protein from plant-based foods if you combine them well and eat a variety.

3. **Myth:** "Protein is only for athletes and bodybuilders."
   **Truth:** Everyone needs protein for healthy muscles, organs, and body systems.

## The Link Between Protein and Feeling Full

Protein can help you feel satisfied after meals. When combined with fiber (from fruits, vegetables, and whole grains), it can keep you feeling comfortable for longer. This can prevent mindless snacking on sugary or salty foods that do not benefit your body. If you notice you are often hungry between meals, adding a bit more protein at breakfast or lunch might help.

## Day-to-Day Protein Examples

- **Breakfast:** Scrambled eggs with spinach, or oatmeal with a spoonful of peanut butter.

- **Snack:** Greek yogurt with berries, or a small handful of almonds.

- **Lunch:** Whole-grain wrap with chicken or tofu, plus vegetables.

- **Dinner:** Salmon with brown rice and steamed broccoli.

- **Dessert (Optional):** A small serving of cottage cheese with fruit, or a glass of low-fat milk.

## Protein for Different Life Stages

- **Children:** Need protein for growth. Beans, lean meats, dairy, and eggs can all help.

- **Teens:** Often have an increased need because they are growing quickly. They also might be involved in sports.

- **Adults:** Use protein to maintain muscle mass. As people age, muscles may weaken, so protein becomes important to reduce muscle loss.

- **Older Adults:** Need to keep protein intake steady to maintain strength and aid recovery from illness.

## Checking for Allergies

Some protein sources cause allergies in some people. Peanuts, eggs, and some seafood are common allergens. If you feel itchy or have other symptoms after eating these foods, you should tell a trusted adult. There are many protein options, so if someone is allergic to peanuts, they could have almonds, pumpkin seeds, or other choices.

## Role of Protein in Healing

If you get injured, your body needs to fix tissues. Proteins provide the foundation for that repair. This is why people recovering from injuries or surgeries are often told to eat enough protein. It gives the body the tools it needs to replace or repair damaged cells.

## Planning Protein-Rich Meals without Overdoing It

1. **Use a palm-sized portion of meat or fish:** This is a simple measure for one serving.

2. **Choose more plant-based proteins during the week:** This adds fiber and can be easier on the budget.

3. **Watch out for too many processed meats:** Bacon, sausage, and hot dogs often have extra salt and preservatives.

4. **Balance your plate:** Add plenty of vegetables or fruits and a whole-grain side. This ensures that protein is part of the meal, not the entire meal.

## Protein Labels and Claims

Some products advertise "added protein" or "high protein." Always check the label to see how much protein is really there and whether the product is healthy overall. A candy bar might say it has added protein, but it could also have a lot of sugar and unhealthy fats. Look at the full nutrition facts, not just the protein number.

# CHAPTER 4

## Carbohydrates: Fuel for Active Days

Carbohydrates, often called "carbs," are one of the main types of nutrients that give your body energy. Think of them like fuel for a car. Without enough carbs, your body might feel tired or lack the quick boost you need for running, jumping, or playing. But not all carbs are the same, and picking the right ones can help you feel your best.

## What Are Carbohydrates?

Carbohydrates are molecules made of carbon, hydrogen, and oxygen. When you eat carbs, your body turns them into glucose, a form of sugar that cells use for energy. Some carbs are broken down quickly, giving you a fast burst of energy. Others break down more slowly, giving a steady supply of energy.

## Types of Carbohydrates

1. **Sugars (Simple Carbohydrates):** These are found in sweets, soda, candy, and also in fruits (natural sugars). Because they break down fast, they can give a quick spike in energy. But if you eat too many added sugars, you might feel a crash later.

2. **Starches (Complex Carbohydrates):** These are found in foods like bread, pasta, rice, and potatoes. They break down more slowly than simple sugars, giving you longer-lasting energy.

3. **Fiber:** A special type of carbohydrate that your body cannot completely break down. Fiber helps with digestion and keeps you full. It also supports healthy gut bacteria and can help control blood sugar levels.

## Why Carbs Are Important

1. **Primary Energy Source:** When you do anything active, from sports to daily chores, carbs often provide the first fuel.

2. **Brain Function:** Your brain uses glucose for power. If you skip carbs entirely, you may feel foggy or have a hard time focusing.

3. **Protects Protein:** When you eat enough carbs, your body does not have to break down protein for energy. This leaves protein free to fix tissues and support other functions.

## Simple Carbs vs. Complex Carbs

- **Simple Carbs:** Candies, sugary cereals, and sugary drinks have lots of simple carbs. Fruit also has simple carbs, but fruit contains fiber and vitamins that help slow sugar absorption.

- **Complex Carbs:** Whole-grain breads, oatmeal, brown rice, and beans give a steady release of energy and are often high in nutrients.

In general, you want more of your carbs to be complex, but that does not mean you can never have sweets. The key is to keep sweets in smaller amounts.

## Whole Grains for Lasting Energy

Whole grains include all parts of the grain kernel: the bran, germ, and endosperm. This means you get fiber, vitamins, and minerals that help your body. Examples:

- **Whole Wheat Bread:** More fiber and nutrients compared to white bread.

- **Brown Rice:** Has more nutrients than white rice.

- **Oats:** Can help lower certain health risks due to their soluble fiber.

- **Quinoa:** A grain-like seed that is also a source of protein.

When you pick whole grains, you support stable energy levels and keep your digestion in better shape.

## The Importance of Fiber

Fiber helps keep your digestive system regular, which can prevent constipation. It also helps control blood sugar by slowing how fast your body absorbs carbs. This can keep you from feeling a sudden rush of energy followed by a crash. Fruits, vegetables, whole grains, beans, and lentils are all good sources of fiber.

## How Many Carbs Do You Need?

The exact amount depends on your age, weight, and how active you are. Most balanced diets have a decent portion of calories from carbs, often around 45-65%. If you do a lot of sports or physical activities, you might need more. If you mostly sit all day, you might need less. Pay attention to how your body feels. If you are always tired or lacking energy, you might need to check the carbs you are eating.

## Good Sources of Carbs

1. **Fruits:** Apples, bananas, berries, oranges, etc. These have natural sugars, fiber, and vitamins.

2. **Vegetables:** Potatoes, peas, corn, and other starchy veggies offer carbs. Even non-starchy veggies have some carbs, although less.

3. **Whole Grains:** Oatmeal, whole wheat pasta, brown rice, barley, and more.

4. **Legumes:** Beans, lentils, and chickpeas have carbs plus protein and fiber.

## Foods High in Added Sugar

Candy bars, cookies, sugary drinks, and pastries have a lot of added sugar. They might taste good, but they do not provide many vitamins or minerals. They give a quick boost of energy, but it does not last. Often, you end up feeling tired later. Eating too many sweets can also lead to weight problems and other issues if repeated over time.

## Balanced Meals with Carbs

A balanced meal has a protein source, a portion of carbs, and some vegetables or fruits. For example:

- **Breakfast:** Oatmeal topped with berries and a side of scrambled eggs.

- **Lunch:** Whole wheat sandwich with lean protein and veggies.

- **Dinner:** Brown rice with chicken (or beans) and mixed vegetables.

You could add healthy fats like avocado or nuts. This kind of balance helps keep your energy steady and provides different nutrients at once.

## Carbs and Physical Activity

If you play sports or do intense exercise, carbs are important. Before a workout, you need carbs for energy. After a workout, some carbs can help refill the energy stores in your muscles. That is why many athletes have snacks like fruit or a sandwich after training. But they also include protein to help muscles recover.

## The Trouble with Too Few Carbs

Some people think cutting out carbs completely is good. However, without enough carbs, you might feel weak, and your body could break down proteins for energy. That can affect muscle building and repair. Also, carbs come packaged with fiber, vitamins, and minerals, especially if you pick whole foods like fruits, vegetables, and whole grains. Missing these can lead to nutrient shortages.

## Healthy Swaps to Reduce Sugary Carbs

1. **Drink Water or Unsweetened Tea:** Replace soda or fruit punch with water.

2. **Pick Whole Fruit instead of Juice:** Whole fruit has fiber that juice does not.

3. **Choose Whole Wheat Bread:** Skip white bread for sandwiches.

4. **Try Sweet Potatoes instead of Regular Fries:** They often have more vitamins and fiber.

## Reading Food Labels for Carbs

When you look at a nutrition label, you will see "Total Carbohydrates," which includes fiber, sugars (both natural and added), and starches. Below that, you might see "Added Sugars," which tells you how much sugar was put in during processing. The higher this number, the less healthy the product might be. Compare products and pick the ones with lower added sugars and higher fiber.

## Glycemic Index (GI) and Glycemic Load (GL)

The glycemic index measures how quickly a food raises your blood sugar. Foods high on the index, like white bread or candy, can cause a fast spike. Foods lower on the index, like whole grains or beans, cause a slower rise, giving more stable energy. The glycemic load also considers the serving size. These tools can be handy, but you do not need to live by them. Simply aiming for more whole foods and fewer heavily processed items often leads to better blood sugar control.

## Carbs and Weight

Eating carbs does not automatically make you gain weight. Extra calories from any source (carbs, proteins, or fats) can cause weight gain if you eat more than your body needs. The problem is that many high-carb foods also have lots of added fats or sugars. If you pick healthier carbs like brown rice, oatmeal, or fruits, and watch portion sizes, you can keep a balanced weight.

## Tips for Packing Carb-Rich Lunches

1. **Whole Grain Sandwiches:** Fill with lean protein, cheese, or a nut spread. Add lettuce, tomato, or other veggies.

2. **Pasta Salad with Veggies:** Use whole wheat pasta and add peppers, cucumbers, and a light dressing.

3. **Rice Bowls:** Brown rice plus beans or tofu, topped with a little salsa or sauce.

4. **Leftover Favorites:** If you have leftover whole grain pizza or a vegetable stir-fry, pack it for the next day.

## Meal Planning for Steady Energy

To keep your body fueled, try to have balanced meals throughout the day. If you skip breakfast, you might feel super hungry later and overeat sugary snacks. If you have a long gap between lunch and dinner, you might look for quick fixes like chips. Small, balanced snacks can help in these gaps. For instance, an apple with peanut butter gives you carbs, protein, and healthy fats all in one snack.

## The Role of Fiber in Carbohydrate Foods

Fiber helps slow down how fast your body absorbs sugar. This stops big spikes in blood sugar, which can lead to crashes later. Fiber also helps you feel full, so you do not get hungry too soon. Good fiber sources include beans, peas, lentils, oats, barley, many fruits, and vegetables like broccoli or Brussels sprouts. Drinking enough water helps fiber do its job better.

## Listening to Your Body

If you eat a sugary snack and feel an energy crash later, that is your body telling you something. Try switching to a piece of fruit or whole-grain toast with a little peanut butter and see if you feel better. Notice how different carbs affect you. Everyone's body reacts a bit differently, so it can help to pay attention and learn from experience.

# Carbohydrate Myths

1. **Myth:** "All carbs are bad."
   **Truth:** Whole carbs like whole grains, fruits, and vegetables are full of nutrients. It is mostly the refined sugars and flours that you should limit.

2. **Myth:** "Carbs make you gain weight quickly."
   **Truth:** Weight gain happens when you eat more calories than you burn, no matter if they come from carbs, fats, or proteins. Healthy carb choices in the right amounts can fit in most diets.

3. **Myth:** "You must avoid bread to be healthy."
   **Truth:** Whole-grain bread can be part of a healthy diet. White bread is less nutritious, but that does not mean you have to avoid it forever. It is just good to include more whole grains overall.

# Handling Cravings for Sugary Foods

Cravings can happen if you are used to having sweets often. Instead of cutting them out fully, try to switch to healthier choices step by step. For example, if you usually drink a can of soda each day, switch to water or a low-sugar drink for a few days a week. Over time, you might find you do not want as much sugar. You can also try sweet fruits, like berries or peaches, to satisfy your taste for sweetness in a healthier way.

# Smart Snacking with Carbs

If you need a snack during a busy day, pick something with fiber and a bit of protein. Examples:

- **Apple or Banana with Peanut Butter**

- **Whole-Grain Crackers with Cheese**

- **Yogurt with Berries**

- **Homemade Trail Mix (Nuts, Seeds, Dry Whole-Grain Cereal)**

These choices give you a slow release of energy instead of a sugar rush.

## Cultural and Festive Carbohydrate Foods

Carbs come in many shapes and forms around the world. From rice dishes in Asia to tortillas in Latin America, to different types of pasta in Italy, you will see carbs as a big part of many diets. Celebrations often include special breads, pastries, or sweet treats. Enjoying these is part of life, and that is fine. Just try not to let these foods replace more balanced meals regularly.

## Carbs for Different Age Groups

- **Children:** Need carbs for growth and energy to play. Whole grains and fruits are great options.

- **Teens:** Often very active with sports or hobbies. They might need more carbs, especially complex carbs.

- **Adults:** Need carbs to keep energy levels steady for work or family life.

- **Older Adults:** Still need carbs, but portion sizes might change if they are less active.

## Storing and Preparing Carbohydrate-Rich Foods

- **Keep Whole Grains Fresh:** Store them in airtight containers to avoid bugs or moisture.

- **Batch Cooking:** Cook a large pot of brown rice or whole wheat pasta to use throughout the week.

- **Freezing Bread:** If you buy more bread than you can use in a few days, freeze some to keep it fresh.

- **Washing and Cutting Fruits:** Prepping fruits ahead of time can make it easier to pick them as a snack instead of cookies.

## Conclusion of Chapter 4

Carbohydrates are the main source of fuel for your body and brain. Picking healthier forms, like whole grains, fruits, and vegetables, can give you steady energy and important nutrients. While sugary treats can be enjoyed sometimes, too much sugar can lead to highs and lows in energy. By learning how different carbs work, you can choose options that keep you feeling your best and support your daily activities. Remember to listen to your body, watch out for signs of energy crashes, and choose carb sources that provide vitamins, minerals, and fiber.

# CHAPTER 5

## Fats: Importance of Healthy Sources

Fats are often misunderstood. Some people think that all fats are bad, while others may eat foods high in fat without knowing how it affects their bodies. The truth is, your body does need certain types of fats. However, it is important to pick the right ones and avoid eating too many of the unhealthy kinds. Fats play a big part in how your body works, from helping you absorb vitamins to keeping your cells functioning properly.

## What Are Fats?

Fats are nutrients found in many foods. Like carbohydrates and proteins, fats provide energy. But they do more than just give you fuel. They help your body absorb certain vitamins, keep your skin and hair healthy, and support the production of important hormones. Fats are made of fatty acids, which can be shaped differently depending on where they come from. Some shapes are better for you than others.

## Why We Need Some Fat

1. **Energy Storage:** When your body takes in more energy (calories) than it needs right away, it stores that energy as fat. This stored fat can be used later if you do not eat enough food to meet your energy demands.

2. **Protecting Organs:** Fat helps pad and protect important organs inside your body.

3. **Vitamin Absorption:** Vitamins A, D, E, and K dissolve in fat. If you do not eat enough healthy fats, your body may not absorb these vitamins well.

4. **Hormone Production:** Your body makes certain hormones with the help of fats. Hormones send signals that keep your body processes in balance.

5. **Keeping You Warm:** Fat under your skin provides insulation and helps you stay warm in cold weather.

## Different Types of Fats

Not all fats affect your body in the same way. Some can benefit you, while others can cause problems if you eat too much of them.

1. **Unsaturated Fats (Good Fats):**

    - **Monounsaturated Fats:** Found in foods like olive oil, avocados, and many nuts. They can help keep your heart healthy.

    - **Polyunsaturated Fats:** Found in foods like salmon, sardines, and walnuts. They contain omega-3 fatty acids that help your brain and heart.

2. **Saturated Fats:**

    - Often found in foods like butter, fatty meats, and some dairy products. Having too many saturated fats can cause concerns for your heart and overall health if you eat them in large amounts regularly.

3. **Trans Fats (Mostly Unhealthy Fats):**

    - These are found in some packaged snacks, baked goods, or fried foods. They are made through a process that changes liquid oils into solid fats. Trans fats are often considered the most harmful type and should be avoided or limited as much as possible.

## How Fats Help the Body

- **Cell Function:** Each cell in your body is surrounded by a layer that contains fats. This layer keeps the cell stable and helps control what goes in and out.

- **Brain Support:** Your brain is made up of a lot of fat. Some healthy fats help with brain development and function.

- **Healthy Skin and Hair:** Fats help keep your skin smooth and your hair strong. If you do not get enough, your skin might get dry or your hair might become dull.

## Daily Fat Needs

The amount of fat you need depends on factors like age, body size, and how active you are. Some general guidelines say that fats should make up around 20-35% of your daily calories. The key is choosing mostly unsaturated fats rather than saturated or trans fats. If you focus on a balanced diet that includes lean proteins, whole grains, fruits, and vegetables, you usually get a healthy range of fats without needing to calculate exact numbers.

## Sources of Healthy Fats

1. **Avocados:** They have monounsaturated fats, fiber, and several vitamins. Avocados can be used in sandwiches, salads, or even smoothies.

2. **Nuts and Seeds:** Almonds, walnuts, chia seeds, and flaxseeds have good fats, protein, and fiber. They make easy snacks or can be sprinkled on dishes.

3. **Fatty Fish:** Salmon, trout, and sardines have omega-3 fatty acids that may help your heart and brain.

4. **Olive Oil:** A common cooking oil with monounsaturated fats that can be healthier than butter.

5. **Peanut Butter or Nut Butters:** Look for natural versions without added sugar or trans fats.

## Reducing Unhealthy Fats

1. **Limit Fried Foods:** Foods deep-fried in oil often absorb a lot of that oil, which can be high in unhealthy fats. If you want fries, baking them at home can be a better choice.

2. **Choose Lean Cuts of Meat:** If you eat meat, look for cuts with less visible fat. Trim off extra fat before cooking.

3. **Check Labels for Trans Fats:** Some packaging might say "partially hydrogenated oil." That is another term for trans fats. Avoid these when possible.

4. **Moderate Your Dairy Intake:** Whole milk, butter, and full-fat cheese are high in saturated fats. You do not have to skip them entirely, but it can help to switch to lower-fat versions or reduce how much you use.

## How Too Much Bad Fat Affects the Body

If you eat large amounts of saturated and trans fats over a long time, you might face these issues:

- **Weight Problems:** Extra fat from unhealthy sources can lead to taking in too many calories, which may cause extra weight.

- **Heart Strain:** High levels of certain fats can affect cholesterol in your blood. This can be risky for your heart and blood vessels.

- **Lack of Nutrients:** If you fill up on fatty, processed foods, you might not have room for fruits, vegetables, and whole grains that provide important vitamins and minerals.

## Balancing Fats with Other Nutrients

While fats are important, do not forget about proteins, carbohydrates, vitamins, and minerals. A balanced meal might have a healthy fat source (like a handful of nuts or a drizzle of olive oil), a protein source (like beans, chicken, or fish), and carbs that have fiber (like whole grains or vegetables). This balance helps your body get everything it needs without overloading on any one nutrient.

## Cooking Tips to Use Healthier Fats

- **Use Olive Oil or Canola Oil:** These have more unsaturated fats than butter.

- **Bake or Grill Instead of Frying:** You can still get crunchy textures by baking with a light coating of oil. Grilling also uses less oil.

- **Add Avocado Slices:** Rather than cheese or mayonnaise, adding avocado can provide creaminess along with good fats.

- **Experiment with Herbs and Spices:** They add flavor without needing too much oil or butter.

## Avoiding Hidden Fats

Foods like doughnuts, cookies, and pastries might have more fat than you realize. Some crackers or microwave popcorn can also have added fats. Read the ingredient list and check for oils that might be high in saturated or trans fats. Even if a label says "0 g trans fat," it can still have a small amount per serving. If the ingredients list "partially hydrogenated oil," that means there are some trans fats in it.

## Myths about Fat

1. **Myth:** "All fats are bad."
   **Truth:** Your body needs certain fats to function. The main issue is eating too much saturated and trans fat.

2. **Myth:** "Foods labeled 'low fat' are always better."
   **Truth:** Some low-fat products have extra sugar or chemicals to improve taste. It is important to check the full label.

3. **Myth:** "Eating fat always leads to weight gain."
   **Truth:** Weight gain happens when you eat more calories than you use. The source can be fats, carbs, or proteins. Healthy fats, in proper amounts, do not automatically cause weight gain.

## Ways to Include Healthy Fats Every Day

- **Smoothies:** Add a spoonful of peanut butter or a slice of avocado for healthy fats.

- **Snacks:** Nuts or seeds can replace chips and other fried snacks.

- **Meals:** Prepare salads with an olive oil-based dressing. Top with a small number of nuts or seeds.

- **Spreads:** Use mashed avocado or hummus on sandwiches instead of mayonnaise or butter.

## Recognizing High-Fat Foods

Some foods are clearly high in fat, like fried chicken or buttered popcorn. Others might be less obvious. Certain kinds of granola bars can have oils high in saturated fats. Muffins or other baked goods often use butter or shortening. Checking labels for saturated or trans fats is a good way to spot which foods to enjoy only in small amounts.

## Fats for Different Ages

1. **Children:** They need some healthy fats for brain growth. Whole milk is often recommended for very young kids, but as they grow, lower-fat dairy can be introduced.

2. **Teens:** Their bodies are changing quickly, so they need enough fat for hormone production. Choosing mostly unsaturated fats is still best.

3. **Adults:** Should watch their intake of saturated and trans fats to support heart health. Unsaturated fats from fish and plants can be helpful.

4. **Older Adults:** Need healthy fats for continued heart and brain support. Lowering saturated and trans fats can help prevent problems.

## Tips for Eating Out

Restaurants often use more oil, butter, or creamy sauces than you might at home. To reduce unhealthy fat intake when dining out:

- Pick grilled or baked options instead of fried items.

- Ask for dressings or sauces on the side.

- Consider sharing large portions or taking half home, so you do not overeat.

- Choose vegetable-based sides instead of fries or onion rings most of the time.

## Healthy Fat in Cultural Foods

Many traditional dishes around the world use healthy fat sources. For example, Mediterranean meals often feature olive oil, nuts, and fish. Japanese meals may include fatty fish like salmon. Some South American dishes use avocados or peanuts in their recipes. Exploring these options can be a tasty way to add good fats into your diet.

## Being Careful with Fat-Free Trends

Years ago, there was a big push for fat-free or low-fat foods. Some of these items replaced fat with extra sugar or salt. A product might say "fat-free," but if it has added sugar, it can still be unhealthy. That is why reading labels and checking the overall nutrition is important. Aim for whole foods that naturally have healthy fats, rather than processed products with long ingredient lists.

## Storing Foods with Fats

- **Nuts and Seeds:** Keep them in a cool, dry place. Some types can go bad if left in a warm spot for too long.

- **Oils:** Most cooking oils are best stored in a dark, cool area. Olive oil can be sensitive to light and heat.

- **Avocados:** Ripen them at room temperature. Once they are soft, store them in the fridge to keep them from spoiling too fast.

- **Fatty Fish:** Freeze it if you are not planning to eat it soon. Thaw it in the fridge when you are ready to cook.

## Balancing Flavor and Health

A small amount of butter or cheese can add taste. The idea is not to give up these flavors entirely but to be careful with how much you use. If your meal includes a heavier sauce or cheese, you might skip adding more fats like cream or extra butter. Balancing helps you enjoy tasty foods without going overboard.

## Conclusion of Chapter 5

Fats are a necessary part of your diet, giving you energy, helping you absorb vitamins, and supporting many body functions. The key is knowing which fats help you and which ones might hurt you if you eat too much. By focusing on unsaturated fats from foods like avocados, nuts, seeds, and certain fish, you can keep your body strong and support a healthy heart and brain. Avoiding or limiting trans fats and being mindful of saturated fats are steps toward better health. With a balanced approach, fats can be a tasty and helpful part of your meals every day.

# CHAPTER 6

## Vitamins: Tiny Helpers for Big Needs

Vitamins are small but mighty. They are often called "micronutrients" because your body only needs them in small amounts, yet they are important for keeping you healthy. They help your body use energy from foods, fix body tissues, and fight off sickness. If you miss certain vitamins for too long, you can feel weak or face other health problems. This chapter will introduce the main vitamins and show you how to get them from foods.

## What Are Vitamins?

Vitamins are chemical compounds that your body cannot make enough of on its own (or at all), so you need to get them from the foods you eat. Each vitamin has special jobs, from helping your eyes see well at night to supporting the way your blood clots if you get a cut. Vitamins work best when you have them in the right amounts, not too little and not too much.

## Different Types of Vitamins

There are many vitamins, but the main ones are usually grouped as follows:

1. **Fat-Soluble Vitamins:** These include vitamins A, D, E, and K. They dissolve in fat, so your body can store them in your liver and fatty tissues.

2. **Water-Soluble Vitamins:** These include vitamin C and the B vitamins (like B1, B2, B3, B6, B9, and B12). Your body cannot store most of these for a long time, so you need to get them more frequently.

## Vitamin A

- **What It Does:** Supports good vision, especially in low light. Also helps your immune system and keeps skin healthy.

- **Where to Find It:** Carrots, sweet potatoes, spinach, kale, and eggs. Orange and dark green vegetables are usually high in vitamin A.

- **Deficiency Issues:** Night blindness (trouble seeing in dim light), dry eyes, or weak immune function.

## Vitamin D

- **What It Does:** Helps your body use calcium to build and maintain strong bones. Also supports your immune system and mood.

- **Where to Find It:** Fatty fish (like salmon, mackerel), egg yolks, and fortified milk or cereals. Your body can also make vitamin D when your skin is in sunlight, but be careful not to get too much sun exposure without protection.

- **Deficiency Issues:** Weak bones, feeling tired, or mood changes. In children, severe deficiency might lead to rickets, where bones become soft or bent.

## Vitamin E

- **What It Does:** Acts as an antioxidant, protecting your cells from damage. Supports your immune system and helps maintain healthy skin and eyes.

- **Where to Find It:** Nuts, seeds, vegetable oils, spinach, and broccoli.

- **Deficiency Issues:** Rare in healthy people, but can include nerve and muscle problems if levels are too low for a long time.

## Vitamin K

- **What It Does:** Helps your blood clot properly, so you stop bleeding if you get a cut. Also supports bone health.

- **Where to Find It:** Leafy greens like kale, spinach, broccoli, and some vegetable oils.

- **Deficiency Issues:** Easy bruising or bleeding more than normal.

## Vitamin C

- **What It Does:** Helps make collagen, which is a part of skin and other tissues. Boosts your immune system and acts as an antioxidant.

- **Where to Find It:** Citrus fruits (like oranges, lemons), strawberries, bell peppers, and tomatoes.

- **Deficiency Issues:** Bleeding gums, slow wound healing, and a condition called scurvy if you have almost no vitamin C.

## B Vitamins

There are several B vitamins, each with its own role:

- **Vitamin B1 (Thiamin):** Helps turn the foods you eat into energy and supports nerve function. Found in whole grains, beans, and pork.

- **Vitamin B2 (Riboflavin):** Assists in energy production and cell growth. Found in milk, eggs, almonds, and spinach.

- **Vitamin B3 (Niacin):** Helps your body use proteins and fats and supports skin health. Found in poultry, fish, and peanuts.

- **Vitamin B6 (Pyridoxine):** Helps your body use and store energy from proteins and carbs. Found in chickpeas, bananas, and salmon.

- **Vitamin B9 (Folate or Folic Acid):** Important for making new cells and DNA. Found in leafy greens, beans, and oranges.

- **Vitamin B12 (Cobalamin):** Helps keep nerves and blood cells healthy and supports making DNA. Found in fish, meat, dairy, and fortified cereals. People who do not eat animal products often need to look for B12-fortified foods or supplements.

## Signs You May Be Missing Vitamins

If you do not get enough of certain vitamins, you may notice signs like:

- Feeling tired or weak more often.

- Dry or irritated skin.

- Trouble healing from small cuts or bruises.

- Problems with vision in dim light.

- Frequent colds or sickness due to a weak immune system.

However, these signs can also be caused by other issues. If you think you are missing vitamins, it helps to check your overall diet or talk to a health professional.

## Getting Vitamins from Food

The best way to get vitamins is through eating a variety of foods. When you eat fruits, vegetables, whole grains, and protein sources, you also get fiber, minerals, and other helpful nutrients along with vitamins. For example, an orange does not just have vitamin C; it also has fiber and other plant compounds that help your body in different ways.

## Supplements: Yes or No?

Many people wonder if they should take vitamin pills or gummies. While supplements can help in some cases—especially if you have a deficiency—most healthy individuals can get the vitamins they need from food. If you think you might be missing certain vitamins, it is best to talk to a health professional rather than starting a supplement on your own. Taking too many supplements can cause problems because vitamins like A, D, E, and K can build up in your body.

## Balancing Vitamins in Meals

One easy method to get a range of vitamins is to eat many different colors of fruits and vegetables. Think of a rainbow on your plate:

- **Red (Tomatoes, Red Peppers):** Often have vitamins A and C.

- **Orange or Yellow (Carrots, Squash):** Can have vitamin A and other antioxidants.

- **Green (Spinach, Broccoli):** Usually high in vitamins K, C, and some B vitamins.

- **Blue or Purple (Eggplant, Blueberries):** Might have antioxidants that help cells.

By having multiple colors, you cover more vitamin bases in a natural way.

## Cooking and Vitamin Loss

Some vitamins can break down when exposed to heat, air, or water. For example, vitamin C can be lost if you boil vegetables for a long time. To keep more vitamins in your foods:

- Steam or stir-fry vegetables instead of boiling them in a large pot of water.

- Use as little water as possible if you do boil.

- Eat some fruits and vegetables raw, like in salads or as snacks.

- Store produce properly, in cool and dark conditions when possible.

## Myths about Vitamins

1. **Myth:** "Taking more vitamins gives you more energy."
   **Truth:** Vitamins help your body use energy, but they do not directly provide energy like calories do. Too many can actually be harmful.

2. **Myth:** "You cannot get enough vitamins from food alone."
   **Truth:** Many people can get everything they need from a varied diet. Supplements can help if there is a real shortage, but they are not always required.

3. **Myth:** "All vitamin supplements are the same."
   **Truth:** Quality can differ, and some might have unnecessary fillers or very high doses. That is why talking to a health professional is wise before taking them.

## Water-Soluble vs. Fat-Soluble Reminders

- **Water-Soluble (Vitamin C and B Vitamins):** Your body does not store them for a long time, so you should eat them more often. They dissolve in water, and extra amounts usually leave the body through urine.

- **Fat-Soluble (Vitamins A, D, E, K):** Your body stores them in fat cells and the liver. Getting too much of these can lead to problems since they do not leave the body quickly.

## Getting Kids Interested in Vitamins

1. **Colorful Plates:** Children are often drawn to bright, varied colors. Offer carrots, bell peppers, blueberries, or kiwi.

2. **Fun Shapes:** Try cutting fruits and veggies into fun shapes or arrange them in a friendly pattern on a plate.

3. **Smoothies:** Blend different fruits and veggies together with yogurt or milk to make a tasty drink full of vitamins.

4. **Get Them Involved:** Let them choose a vegetable at the store or help wash it before cooking. This can make them more curious about what they eat.

## When to Be Careful

- **Allergies or Food Limits:** If you avoid dairy or animal products, watch out for possible shortages of vitamins like B12 or D.

- **Picky Eating:** If someone eats only a few types of food, they might miss vitamins that come from other sources.

- **Excessive Supplement Use:** More is not always better. Some vitamins can build up to harmful levels.

## Examples of Vitamin-Rich Meals

1. **Breakfast:** Whole-grain cereal with milk (vitamins B and D, if the milk is fortified), plus berries (vitamin C) on top.

2. **Lunch:** Spinach salad with chicken or beans, peppers, and a light dressing (vitamins A, C, and K, plus some B vitamins).

3. **Snack:** An orange or a handful of strawberries (vitamin C).

4. **Dinner:** Salmon with roasted broccoli and sweet potato (vitamin D from salmon, vitamins A and C from veggies).

Remember, adding a small amount of healthy fat to your vegetables can help your body absorb vitamins A, D, E, and K more easily.

## Possible Signs of Too Many Vitamins

While not common from food alone, having too many vitamin supplements can lead to problems:

- **Vitamin A Overdose:** Can cause headaches, dizziness, or even damage organs if it is very high over time.

- **Vitamin D Overdose:** Might lead to raised calcium levels, which can harm kidneys.

- **Vitamin E Overdose:** Could interfere with blood clotting.

That is why it is safer to eat a balanced diet and be thoughtful about supplements.

## Storing Vitamins and Food

- **Eat Fresh Produce Soon:** Vitamins can break down over time. Buy smaller amounts more often if possible.

- **Keep Frozen Options:** Frozen fruits and vegetables can be nearly as nutritious as fresh ones, and they last longer.

- **Avoid High Heat or Sunlight:** Some vitamins, like vitamin C, break down faster in heat or sunlight.

## Conclusion of Chapter 6

Vitamins might be small, but they help your body work properly in many ways, from keeping your eyes sharp to boosting your immune system. By eating a variety of fruits, vegetables, whole grains, and protein sources, you can get most or all of the vitamins you need. Pay attention to both fat-soluble and water-soluble vitamins, and remember that real food is usually the best source. Supplements can be helpful in certain cases, but they are not a cure-all for poor eating habits. With an awareness of where vitamins come from and how they benefit you, you can enjoy colorful, balanced meals that keep your body strong and healthy.

# CHAPTER 7

## Minerals: Key to Supporting Your Body

Minerals are like little helpers that keep your body working properly. You might not think about them as often as proteins, carbs, or fats, but they are just as important. They support your bones, help your nerves send signals, keep your heart beating, and even help make hormones. This chapter will explain why minerals matter, how they work in your body, and the many foods you can eat to get them.

## What Are Minerals?

Minerals are elements that come from the earth. They are in the soil, and plants absorb them. When we eat those plants (or animals that ate those plants), we get the minerals into our bodies. Unlike vitamins, minerals are not made by living things. Instead, they are part of the natural environment. Think of iron, calcium, or potassium. These are all minerals you have probably heard of before.

Your body needs many different kinds of minerals, but it can only store some of them for a short time. Others can be stored for longer. If you do not get enough of a certain mineral, you might feel weak, tired, or develop other health problems. If you get too much of a certain mineral (which is not very common if you are just eating regular foods), that can also cause issues. The key is balance.

## Major Minerals and Trace Minerals

Experts usually split minerals into two main groups:

1. **Major Minerals (Macrominerals)**: These are minerals you need in larger amounts. They include calcium, phosphorus, magnesium, sodium, potassium, chloride, and sometimes sulfur.

2. **Trace Minerals (Microminerals)**: These are minerals you only need in small amounts, but they are still vital. They include iron, zinc, iodine, selenium, copper, manganese, fluoride, and a few others.

Even though you only need tiny amounts of trace minerals, they are still essential for important tasks in your body.

## Why Your Body Needs Minerals

- **Bone and Teeth Health**: Minerals like calcium and phosphorus help build strong bones and teeth.

- **Fluid Balance**: Sodium, potassium, and chloride help your body control the balance of water and fluids inside and outside your cells.

- **Muscle and Nerve Function**: Minerals allow your nerves to send messages, telling your muscles when to move.

- **Oxygen Transport**: Iron is needed to carry oxygen in your blood, helping every part of your body get the oxygen it needs.

- **Immune Support**: Zinc, selenium, and other minerals support your immune system, helping you stay well.

# Calcium

1. **Role in the Body**
   Calcium is the most common mineral in your body. Most of it is stored in your bones and teeth. Your body also uses calcium to help your muscles move and to send signals through nerves. If you do not have enough calcium in your diet, your body may pull calcium out of your bones, making them weaker over time.

2. **Food Sources**

   - Dairy products like milk, yogurt, cheese.
   - Leafy green vegetables like kale and collard greens.
   - Calcium-fortified drinks (some types of orange juice or plant-based milks).
   - Tofu made with calcium sulfate.

3. **Signs of Low Calcium**
   In the short term, you might not notice much, but over time, bones can become weaker (a condition called osteoporosis in adults). Getting enough calcium when you are young helps set a strong base for your bones as you get older.

---

# Phosphorus

1. **Role in the Body**
   Phosphorus works with calcium to build bones and teeth. It also helps your body make energy. Every cell uses phosphorus to do its tasks.

2. **Food Sources**

    - Dairy products, meats, and poultry.

    - Fish like salmon.

    - Nuts, beans, and seeds.

    - Whole grains.

3. **Balance with Calcium**
   Your body keeps calcium and phosphorus in a balanced relationship. Too much of one can affect the other. Luckily, if you eat a typical variety of whole foods, you usually get enough phosphorus without trying too hard.

---

# Magnesium

1. **Role in the Body**
   Magnesium supports muscles and nerve function. It also helps your heart rhythm stay steady and helps your body create proteins. Magnesium is part of more than 300 different actions in your body, which is a lot!

2. **Food Sources**

    - Green leafy vegetables (spinach, Swiss chard).

    - Nuts and seeds (almonds, pumpkin seeds).

    - Whole grains (brown rice, whole wheat bread).

    - Beans and lentils.

3. **Possible Shortages**
   If you do not get enough magnesium, you might feel muscle cramps or feel tired. But serious shortages are less common if you eat a balanced diet with a mix of plant-based foods.

---

# Sodium

1. **Role in the Body**
   Sodium helps control your body's fluid balance. It also helps your nerves send signals. Most people think of sodium as "salt," but salt is actually sodium chloride (a combination of sodium and chloride).

2. **Food Sources**

   - Table salt.

   - Many processed foods (chips, canned soups, fast food) often have high sodium.

   - Bread, cheese, and cured meats can also be high in sodium.

3. **Too Much Sodium**
   While your body needs some sodium, it is easy to get too much, especially from processed foods. Too much sodium can cause your body to hold onto water, which can affect your heart and blood pressure. That is why many people try to limit how much salt they eat.

---

# Potassium

1. **Role in the Body**
   Potassium works together with sodium to balance fluids in and around your cells. It also helps muscles contract and supports normal blood pressure.

2. **Food Sources**

   - Bananas, oranges, melons.
   - Potatoes, beans, peas.
   - Tomatoes and leafy green vegetables.
   - Yogurt and dairy products.

3. **Staying Balanced**
   A shortage of potassium might lead to muscle weakness or cramps. Eating lots of fruits and vegetables usually gives you plenty of potassium.

---

# Chloride

1. **Role in the Body**
   Chloride partners with sodium to help keep your body fluids balanced. It also helps your stomach make acid that breaks down food.

2. **Food Sources**

   - Table salt (sodium chloride).

- Seaweed, tomatoes, and lettuce.
- Many salty foods.

3. **Everyday Balance**
   Since salt is so common, many people get enough chloride without even trying. Just like sodium, too much can be a concern if you rely heavily on processed foods.

---

# Iron

1. **Role in the Body**
   Iron is a key part of hemoglobin, the substance in red blood cells that carries oxygen. Without iron, your cells do not get enough oxygen, and you can feel very tired. Iron also helps with immune support and brain function.

2. **Food Sources**

   - Red meat, poultry, fish.
   - Beans, lentils, tofu, and spinach.
   - Iron-fortified cereals or breads.

3. There are two types of iron in foods: heme iron (mostly in animal foods) and non-heme iron (in plants). Heme iron is absorbed more easily, but vitamin C (from fruits or veggies) can help your body absorb more non-heme iron.

4. **Signs of Low Iron**
   If you do not get enough iron, you might develop anemia, which makes you feel weak and short of breath. Children, teens, and women often need more iron because of growth or other factors.

# Zinc

1. **Role in the Body**
Zinc helps your immune system, wound healing, and many chemical actions in your body. It also plays a part in taste and smell.

2. **Food Sources**

    - Meat, poultry, seafood.
    - Beans, nuts, seeds.
    - Whole grains.
    - Some dairy products.

3. **Shortage Concerns**
Low zinc might lead to slower wound healing or more frequent infections. Getting enough protein from varied sources often provides zinc as well.

---

# Iodine

1. **Role in the Body**
Iodine is needed to make thyroid hormones, which help control how your body uses energy. If you do not get enough iodine, your thyroid gland can become enlarged (forming a goiter).

2. **Food Sources**

    - Iodized salt (table salt with added iodine).

- Seafood like fish and seaweed.
- Dairy from cows that graze on iodine-rich land.

3. **Importance of Iodized Salt**
Many countries add iodine to table salt to help prevent iodine shortages. If you do not use iodized salt, you might need other iodine sources in your meals.

---

# Selenium

1. **Role in the Body**
Selenium works as an antioxidant and helps your immune system. It also helps make thyroid hormones.

2. **Food Sources**
   - Brazil nuts (known for very high selenium).
   - Fish, meat, eggs.
   - Whole grains and seeds (depends on soil content).

3. **Caution with Too Much**
While rare, eating an extreme amount of selenium can cause problems. Most people do not need to worry if they eat a normal range of foods.

---

## Copper, Manganese, Fluoride, and More

- **Copper**: Helps with iron use and red blood cell formation. Found in nuts, seeds, liver, and seafood.

- **Manganese**: Helps enzymes in the body. Found in nuts, whole grains, and leafy vegetables.

- **Fluoride**: Helps keep teeth strong and prevent tooth decay. Often added to public drinking water in some areas. Also found in some seafood and tea.

These trace minerals might sound minor, but they still help keep you healthy. Together, they perform tasks that you might not even notice—until there is a shortage.

---

## Getting Enough Minerals from Food

The best way to get minerals is to eat a mix of foods:

1. **Fruits and Vegetables**: Provide potassium, magnesium, and various trace minerals.

2. **Whole Grains**: Offer magnesium, selenium, and iron (if fortified).

3. **Protein Sources**: Meats, fish, beans, eggs, and nuts give you iron, zinc, and other minerals.

4. **Dairy or Dairy Alternatives**: Supply calcium, phosphorus, and sometimes added vitamin D.

If you rely too much on processed foods, you might get too much sodium and not enough potassium or magnesium. Cooking your own meals at home or choosing less processed options can help you keep minerals in balance.

---

## Possible Problems with Too Many Minerals

It is uncommon to get too many minerals from food alone. But if you take high-dose mineral supplements or eat too many fortified products, you might overdo it. For instance:

- **Too Much Iron** can cause damage to organs over time.

- **Too Much Sodium** can affect your heart and blood pressure.

- **Too Much Fluoride** may lead to spots on teeth or other issues.

Always follow instructions on any supplements, and talk to a professional if you think you need more than the usual amounts.

---

## Signs You May Not Be Getting Enough

- **Tiredness, Weakness**: Could be linked to low iron or magnesium.

- **Muscle Cramps**: Might point to low potassium or magnesium.

- **Frequent Illness**: Low zinc or selenium could impact your immune system.

- **Bone Problems**: Not enough calcium or phosphorus can lead to weak bones over time.

These issues are not always due to mineral shortages, but if they happen often, it might help to check your diet.

## Tips for Keeping Mineral Levels Steady

1. **Eat a Variety of Foods**: Different foods have different minerals. Mixing fruits, vegetables, whole grains, beans, nuts, dairy, meat, or fish can cover your bases.

2. **Check Food Labels**: Some labels show how much calcium, iron, sodium, or potassium are in a serving. This helps you see if something is very high or low in a certain mineral.

3. **Use Herbs and Spices**: To reduce how much salt (sodium) you eat, try herbs and spices for flavor instead of piling on salt.

4. **Consider Fortified Foods**: If you do not get enough of a certain mineral (like iodine or iron), sometimes fortified foods (such as iron-fortified cereal) can help.

## Balancing Minerals for Overall Health

Minerals do not work alone. For example, calcium often pairs with vitamin D to help your bones. Iron is better absorbed when you also eat vitamin C from fruits or vegetables. Potassium helps counterbalance sodium. Think of it as a team effort inside your body. Getting a balanced diet with the right nutrients helps each mineral do its job.

## Real-Life Examples of Mineral-Rich Meals

- **Breakfast**: Whole-grain cereal (iron-fortified) with milk (calcium), plus a banana (potassium).

- **Lunch**: Bean soup (iron, magnesium), side salad (various minerals from veggies), and a slice of whole-grain bread (trace minerals).

- **Snack**: Almonds (magnesium, copper) or yogurt (calcium, phosphorus).

- **Dinner**: Baked salmon (selenium, iodine if sea-caught), roasted broccoli (various minerals), and a small baked potato (potassium).

These choices give you a range of minerals throughout the day.

---

## Caring for Your Minerals: Storage and Cooking

- **Store Fresh Produce Properly**: Fruits and vegetables can lose some mineral content over time, but not as quickly as vitamins might. Still, it is best to store them in a cool place.

- **Avoid Oversoaking Vegetables**: Some minerals can leach into the water. Light steaming or quick stir-frying can keep more minerals in your food.

- **Eating Skins**: For foods like potatoes or apples, the skins often have extra minerals (and fiber). Wash them well first if you plan to eat the peel.

## Myths about Minerals

1. **Myth**: "Only older people need extra calcium."
   **Truth**: Calcium is important at every age. Kids and teens need it for growing bones, while adults need it to maintain bone strength.

2. **Myth**: "If I take a multi-mineral supplement, I do not need to eat well."
   **Truth**: Supplements can help fill gaps, but real foods provide a complex mix of nutrients that work together in ways pills might not.

3. **Myth**: "Salt is always bad."
   **Truth**: Your body needs sodium, but too much from salty snacks and processed meals can cause problems. Moderation is the key.

---

## When to Consider Mineral Supplements

Some people might have specific needs. For example, if you do not eat any animal products, you might need extra iron or zinc from plant-based sources or a supplement. If you have a medical condition that affects absorption, a professional might suggest supplements. But for most healthy people, a balanced diet usually does the job.

---

# CHAPTER 8

## Water: Why Staying Hydrated Matters

Water is one of the simplest and most vital parts of your daily routine. You drink it, wash with it, swim in it, and your body depends on it for almost every function. Without enough water, you can become tired, dizzy, or even seriously ill. Staying hydrated makes sure your cells can do their jobs, your blood flows properly, and your body keeps a steady temperature. This chapter will show why water is so important and how to make sure you drink enough every day.

## Why Water Is Essential

1. **Most of Your Body Is Water**: More than half of your body weight is water. Water is in your blood, cells, and every tissue.

2. **Helps Transport Nutrients**: Water carries vitamins, minerals, and other nutrients to your cells through your bloodstream.

3. **Removes Waste**: Your body uses water to get rid of waste through urine, sweat, and bowel movements.

4. **Temperature Control**: When you are hot, you sweat. As the sweat evaporates, it cools your skin.

5. **Protects Joints and Tissues**: Water helps keep your joints cushioned. It also helps keep sensitive tissues, like your eyes or mouth, moist.

Every cell in your body needs water, which is why going without water for even a single day can make you feel unwell.

## Daily Water Needs

How much water do you need each day? It can vary based on your size, age, and how active you are. A common guideline is around 6 to 8 cups of water a day for adults, but this can include water from foods and other drinks. Kids might need a bit less, while very active teens or adults in hot weather might need more. Rather than counting every drop, you can pay attention to signs in your body:

- If your urine is light yellow or clear, you are likely well hydrated.

- If it is dark yellow, you may need more fluids.

- If you feel thirsty, you should drink water soon. Thirst is a signal that your body already needs fluid.

---

## Sources of Water

1. **Drinking Water**: Straight from the tap or from a water bottle is often the simplest choice.

2. **Foods**: Fruits like watermelon or oranges can have a high water content. Soups or broths also add to your fluid intake.

3. **Other Drinks**: Milk, juice, tea, and even coffee have water, though they can also have sugar or caffeine. It is best not to rely on sugary or caffeinated drinks for most of your water needs.

If your tap water is not safe or has a strong smell, filters or bottled water might be options, but it depends on your local situation.

## Dehydration: When Your Body Lacks Water

Dehydration happens when you lose more water than you take in. You can lose water through sweating, breathing, and using the bathroom. If you do not replace that fluid, problems can occur:

- **Early Signs**: Thirst, dry mouth, feeling tired.

- **Moderate Signs**: Headaches, dizziness, less frequent urination.

- **Severe Signs**: Very dark urine, rapid heartbeat, confusion, or fainting.

Children and older adults are at higher risk because they may not notice thirst as quickly or might forget to drink. Athletes who sweat a lot can also be at risk if they do not drink enough during and after their activities.

---

## Water and Physical Performance

When you exercise, your muscles produce heat. You sweat to cool down. If you do not drink enough water, you cannot sweat effectively, and your body temperature may rise. You might feel weak, tired, or get muscle cramps. Even mild dehydration can reduce your speed or endurance. Drinking water before, during, and after exercise is important to keep your body working at its best.

## Plain Water vs. Sports Drinks

Sports drinks often have electrolytes (like sodium and potassium) and sugar to replace what you lose through sweat. They can be helpful for athletes who do intense workouts for more than an hour at a time. However, for shorter activities or regular daily movement, plain water is usually enough. Sports drinks can have extra sugar and calories you might not need. If you want electrolytes without the sugar, some lower-sugar or no-sugar options exist, but for most people, water alone will do fine unless you are sweating a lot.

---

## Water and the Brain

Staying hydrated supports clear thinking. Your brain is mostly water, so when you do not drink enough, you might have trouble concentrating, feel grumpy, or get a headache. Drinking enough water can help you think more clearly and keep your mood steady. Many students find they can focus better at school if they sip water through the day.

---

## Tips for Drinking More Water

1. **Carry a Water Bottle**: Having water handy makes it easier to sip throughout the day.

2. **Flavor It Naturally**: If you do not like plain water, add slices of citrus fruit, cucumber, or berries.

3. **Set Reminders**: Alarms on your phone or notes on the fridge can remind you to drink.

4. **Drink Water at Meals**: Instead of sweet drinks, have water with your food.

5. **Track Your Cups**: Use a simple chart or an app if you want to be sure you are getting enough.

---

## Different Kinds of Water

- **Tap Water**: In many places, tap water is safe, cheap, and easy to get. Some cities add fluoride to help protect teeth.

- **Bottled Water**: Convenient but can be more expensive and create plastic waste.

- **Filtered Water**: Using a pitcher filter or a filter attached to the faucet can remove certain tastes or contaminants.

- **Mineral Water**: Comes from natural springs and may contain minerals like calcium or magnesium. It can taste different from normal water but is usually more costly.

Pick what works for you, but the goal is to drink enough clean water, whatever the source.

---

## Water in Different Seasons

- **Hot Weather**: You sweat more, so you lose more fluid. Drink water regularly, even before you feel thirsty. Wear light clothes and try to stay in the shade or air-conditioned spaces when it is very hot.

- **Cold Weather**: You may not feel as thirsty, but your body still needs water. Heating indoors can dry out the air, making you lose water through breathing.

- **Rainy or Humid Conditions**: You might still sweat, even if you do not feel very hot. Keep drinking water because your body's cooling system is at work.

## Water and Illness

If you have a fever, you sweat more. If you have vomiting or diarrhea, your body loses even more fluids. In these cases, you need extra water to replace what you lose. Sometimes doctors recommend an oral rehydration solution (like certain store-bought mixes) that has a balance of salts and sugar to help the body absorb water better. This is important for young kids or older people who can become dehydrated quickly.

## How Water Supports Digestion

Water helps break down food so your body can take in the nutrients. It also helps move waste through your intestines. If you do not drink enough, you might get constipated. Fiber needs water to do its job. So if you are eating a high-fiber diet, you also need enough water to help everything pass smoothly.

## Checking Your Water Safety

In many places, tap water is tested to make sure it meets safety rules. If you are unsure, you can check local reports or use a home water test kit. Sometimes well water or water in older buildings can have contaminants. In these cases, a filter or bottled water might be necessary. You can also boil water to kill germs, though boiling does not remove chemicals or heavy metals—it mainly kills bacteria and viruses.

---

## Water vs. Other Beverages

- **Juice**: Can have vitamins but often has a lot of sugar. Diluting juice with water can cut down on sugar.

- **Soda**: Usually has sugar or artificial sweeteners and does not hydrate as well because of the extra ingredients.

- **Tea and Coffee**: Contain water, but also caffeine, which can make you go to the bathroom more often. Moderate amounts can still help with hydration, but plain water is usually the best choice.

- **Milk**: Has water plus protein, calcium, and other nutrients. It is helpful but still has calories you might not need if you drink large amounts.

---

## Fun Ways to Stay Hydrated

1. **Make Fruity Ice Cubes**: Freeze bits of fruit with water in ice trays. They look pretty and add a little flavor.

2. **Create Cool Blends**: Blend watermelon, ice, and a bit of lime juice for a refreshing drink.

3. **Use Fun Cups**: A favorite cup or straw can encourage kids (and grown-ups) to drink more water.

4. **Set a Challenge**: Challenge your family or friends to see who can reach their water goal each day.

---

## Signs You Might Be Drinking Too Much Water

Though it is rare, it is possible to drink too much water, especially in short periods of time. This can upset the balance of sodium in your body. Athletes who drink huge amounts of water without replacing electrolytes can face a condition known as hyponatremia. Symptoms might include confusion or nausea. For most people, this is not a concern, but it is something to be aware of if you consume very large amounts all at once.

---

## Cultural Views on Water

In many parts of the world, drinking water with meals is standard. In others, people may drink tea or other drinks instead of plain water. Some cultures have traditions of offering water to guests as a polite gesture. Understanding these habits can help us see how different people meet their hydration needs.

## Storing and Handling Water

- **Clean Bottles**: If you reuse water bottles, wash them regularly to prevent germs.

- **No Direct Sunlight**: Keeping clear plastic bottles in direct sunlight for a long time can heat the water, and sometimes chemicals might seep out.

- **Refrigerate if Possible**: Cool water can taste fresher and help prevent bacterial growth.

## Water and Weight Management

Sometimes your body can confuse thirst with hunger, making you think you need a snack when a glass of water might have been enough. Drinking water before meals might help you avoid overeating. Also, water has no calories, so replacing sugary drinks with water can cut down on overall calorie intake.

## Children and Hydration

Kids can get busy playing and forget to drink water. Adults can help by:

- Offering water regularly.

- Keeping water bottles within reach.

- Reminding kids to sip water before, during, and after they play, especially if it is hot.

## Traveling Tips

When you travel, especially to places where tap water might not be safe, you can:

- Use sealed bottled water for drinking and brushing teeth.

- Avoid ice in drinks if you are not sure about the water used to make it.

- Stick to cooked foods that are served hot if water safety is a concern.

This helps prevent illnesses linked to contaminated water.

---

## Conclusion of Chapter 8

Water is the simplest and most important nutrient for your body. It helps carry nutrients, remove waste, and keep you cool. If you do not get enough water, you might feel tired, dizzy, or get headaches. The good news is that it is not hard to stay hydrated if you make water a regular part of your day. By sipping water often, choosing fruits and veggies that contain water, and being mindful of your thirst, you can keep your body running at its best. Whether you are an athlete, a student, or just enjoying daily life, water is a friend you do not want to ignore.

# CHAPTER 9

## Creating Balanced Meals

Building a balanced meal is like putting together a puzzle. Each piece is important, and when you fit them together, you get a complete picture. A balanced meal supports your body by providing a good mix of nutrients: proteins, carbohydrates, fats, vitamins, and minerals. It also gives you energy without too much of anything you do not need. In this chapter, we will explore ways to plan and prepare balanced meals that work for different tastes and lifestyles.

## Why Balanced Meals Matter

1. **Steady Energy**
   When you include a variety of foods in a meal, you get a steady release of energy. Balanced meals often have whole grains (for longer-lasting energy), proteins (to help build and fix your body), and a bit of healthy fat (to keep you satisfied). If you only eat one type of food, like a bowl of pasta with no protein or vegetables, you might feel an energy spike and then a sudden drop.

2. **Complete Nutrition**
   Each food group brings its own nutrients. Proteins bring amino acids, whole grains bring fiber, fruits and vegetables bring vitamins and minerals, and healthy fats help you absorb some nutrients. By mixing them, you get a better chance of meeting your nutrition needs each day.

3. **Healthy Weight Maintenance**
   Balanced meals can help you avoid overeating. If you have enough protein, fiber, and healthy fats, you tend to feel satisfied longer. This can reduce snacking on less helpful foods.

4. **Supports Growth and Repair**
   Kids, teens, and adults all need nutrients to keep their bodies in good shape. Balanced meals supply the building blocks for growing taller (when you are young) and keeping muscles, bones, and tissues in good order.

---

## Simple Ways to Organize Your Meals

There are many ways to build a balanced plate, but here is a simple approach you can use:

1. **Fill Half Your Plate with Vegetables and Fruits**
   This helps you get enough vitamins, minerals, and fiber. It can also keep you from eating too many other foods. For example, a mix of carrots, broccoli, and bell peppers or a side of fruit can add color and nutrients.

2. **Use a Quarter of Your Plate for Protein**
   This can be lean meat, fish, beans, lentils, tofu, eggs, or dairy. Protein helps fix and build tissues and keep you feeling satisfied.

3. **Use a Quarter of Your Plate for Whole Grains or Starchy Veggies**
   Brown rice, oatmeal, whole wheat bread, quinoa, or starchy vegetables like potatoes or corn can fit here. These foods give your body energy.

4. **Add a Small Amount of Healthy Fats**

    You can drizzle olive oil on your vegetables, add a few slices of avocado, or sprinkle nuts and seeds on a salad. Healthy fats help you absorb nutrients like vitamins A, D, E, and K.

5. **Drink Water**

    Water is your best friend at mealtime. It helps transport nutrients through your body and keeps you from loading up on sugary drinks.

---

## Building Breakfast

Breakfast can set the tone for your day. If you start with a meal that has both protein and healthy carbohydrates, you might feel more awake and ready to go. Here are a few ideas:

1. **Oatmeal with Toppings**

    - Base: Rolled oats or steel-cut oats.

    - Toppings: Berries, bananas, nuts, or seeds.

    - Extra Protein: A spoonful of peanut butter or a side of scrambled eggs.

2. This option gives you fiber, vitamins, and some protein. The slow-digesting carbs from the oats can keep you feeling full until your next meal.

3. **Egg Scramble with Veggies**

    - Eggs: A good source of protein.

- Veggies: Spinach, tomatoes, onions, peppers.
- Whole Grain Toast: For steady energy.

4. You can top your eggs with a little cheese if you like, but try not to go overboard on added fats. The veggies add color and extra vitamins.

5. **Yogurt and Fruit Parfait**

    - Plain Yogurt: Greek yogurt often has more protein.
    - Layer with Fruits: Strawberries, blueberries, or peaches.
    - Add Crunch: Whole-grain cereal, granola (low sugar), or chopped nuts.

6. This is a simple way to get calcium, vitamins, and fiber. You can control how sweet it is by choosing fresh fruits instead of sugary toppings.

---

## Creating Balanced Lunches

Lunch can be a time to refuel, especially if you have had an active morning or if you plan to do more in the afternoon. Balanced lunches can keep you from feeling so hungry that you end up grabbing junk food later.

1. **Whole Grain Sandwich**

    - Bread: Choose whole wheat or another whole grain.

- Protein: Turkey, chicken, tuna, beans, or hummus.
- Veggies: Lettuce, tomato, cucumbers, spinach, or shredded carrots.
- Extra: A slice of cheese or avocado if you like.

2. Pair it with a small side salad, carrot sticks, or fruit. That way you get vitamins and fiber.

3. **Leftovers from Dinner**
   If you have leftover chicken, beans, or grains, you can repurpose them. Combine them with fresh vegetables to make a quick salad or a simple bowl meal. Just make sure you reheat foods safely, if needed, and add fresh produce or fruit to balance it out.

4. **Soup and Whole Grain Crackers**

   - Soup Base: Choose a broth-based soup instead of a creamy one to limit saturated fat.
   - Add Ins: Lean meat, beans, or lentils for protein; veggies like carrots, celery, and onions for vitamins and minerals.
   - Whole Grain Crackers: For healthy carbs and a bit of extra fiber.

5. This can be comforting and filling, especially on cool days. You can finish with a piece of fruit for sweetness.

# Dinner: Bringing It All Together

Dinner is often the largest meal for many families. It is a chance to sit together and enjoy a variety of foods. However, large does not mean unbalanced. Try these strategies:

1. **One-Pan Meals**
   Bake or roast a mix of lean meat (chicken or fish) with chopped vegetables (broccoli, carrots, zucchini) and a starch (potatoes or sweet potatoes). Season with herbs instead of heavy sauces. This makes cleanup easier and gives you a balanced meal in one dish.

2. **Stir-Fry**
   - Protein: Chicken, tofu, shrimp, or lean beef cut into small pieces.
   - Veggies: Bell peppers, onions, carrots, snap peas, or bok choy.
   - Sauce: A light sauce using low-sodium soy sauce, garlic, and a bit of ginger.
   - Whole Grain Side: Brown rice or whole grain noodles.

3. This dish is quick and allows you to mix many vegetables. Just watch out for sugary or salty bottled sauces.

4. **Pasta with Extras**
   - Noodles: Pick whole wheat pasta for fiber.
   - Sauce: Tomato-based sauce or a lighter olive oil-based sauce.

- Protein: Lean ground turkey, beans, or chicken strips.

- Vegetables: Add chopped spinach, mushrooms, or zucchini into the sauce.

5. This boosts nutrients and fiber. You can top it with a sprinkle of cheese, but do not let the cheese become the main event.

---

## Snacks and Small Meals

Balanced eating does not have to end at your main meals. Snacks can be part of a healthy plan if you choose them well and watch portion sizes.

1. **Fruit with Nut Butter**
   Apples or bananas with peanut butter or almond butter give carbohydrates, fiber, and a bit of protein.

2. **Veggies with Dip**
   Carrots, cucumber slices, or bell pepper strips with hummus or a yogurt-based dip can keep you satisfied without lots of calories.

3. **Nuts and Seeds**
   Almonds, walnuts, or pumpkin seeds provide protein, healthy fats, and some minerals.

4. **Low-Fat Yogurt**
   Offers calcium and protein, especially if you choose a Greek-style yogurt. Aim for options with little or no added sugar.

---

# Planning Meals in Advance

One big challenge for many people is the lack of time. A busy schedule can make it easy to skip balanced meals. That is why planning is so important.

1. **Meal Planning**

    - Write down your meals for the week.
    - Make a shopping list based on those meals.
    - Prep ingredients in advance, like washing vegetables or cooking whole grains in batches.

2. This helps you avoid last-minute fast-food stops.

3. **Batch Cooking**
   Cook a large pot of soup, stew, or chili with lean protein and veggies. Freeze portions in containers. During the week, you just need to heat a portion and pair it with a side salad or whole grain bread.

4. **Overnight Oats or Mason Jar Salads**

    - Overnight Oats: Mix oats, milk (or a milk substitute), and fruit in a jar. Let it sit in the fridge overnight. In the morning, you have a quick meal.
    - Mason Jar Salads: Layer dressing at the bottom, harder vegetables next, and lettuce or greens on top. Store in the fridge, and shake before eating.

## Eating Together and Sharing Responsibility

Families that eat together often find it easier to include fruits, veggies, and healthy proteins. Everyone can join in the meal planning and cooking. This helps children learn about food and may encourage them to try more foods.

- **Involve Kids**: Have them help wash produce or measure ingredients.

- **Set a Good Example**: If grown-ups enjoy balanced meals, kids are more likely to try them too.

- **Talk about the Meal**: Discuss flavors, colors, and textures, making the meal a fun learning experience.

---

## Balancing Different Dietary Choices

Not everyone eats meat, dairy, or certain grains. Whether you are vegetarian, vegan, or have food allergies, you can still build balanced meals with a bit of creativity.

1. **Vegetarian Meals**

    - Protein from beans, lentils, tofu, tempeh, or eggs (if allowed).

    - Plenty of vegetables and fruits.

    - Whole grains like brown rice, quinoa, or whole wheat pasta.

    - Healthy fats from nuts, seeds, or avocado.

2. **Dairy-Free Meals**

    - Use calcium-fortified plant-based milks, such as soy or almond milk.

    - Check labels to ensure you get enough calcium, vitamin D, and other nutrients.

    - Swap cheese with other toppings, like fresh herbs or a drizzle of olive oil for flavor.

3. **Gluten-Free Meals**

    - Instead of wheat, try rice, corn, or gluten-free oats.

    - Beans and potatoes are also good carb sources.

    - Make sure to check product labels because gluten can show up in unexpected places.

---

## Avoiding Too Much Sugar, Salt, or Unhealthy Fat

A balanced meal also means watching out for too many extras:

1. **Sugar**
   Try to flavor meals with herbs, spices, or natural fruit sweetness. Reserve desserts or sweet treats for special times or in small amounts.

2. **Salt (Sodium)**
   Use herbs, garlic, onions, lemon, or vinegar for flavor instead of salt. You can add a small pinch of salt while cooking but avoid adding lots at the table.

3. **Unhealthy Fats**
   Keep fried foods to a minimum. Instead, bake, grill, or stir-fry with less oil. Choose healthy oils (like olive or canola) and use them sparingly.

## Overcoming Common Obstacles

1. **Busy Schedules**
   If you do not have time to cook every day, prep ahead. Use weekends or free evenings to cook in batches or pre-chop veggies.

2. **Picky Eaters**
   Offer a variety of foods in small portions. Let children pick which veggie they want to try. Keep introducing new options without pressure.

3. **Limited Kitchen Skills**
   Start with simple meals: stir-fry, baked chicken, or a basic soup. Follow easy recipes and learn as you go. Over time, you will become more confident.

## Sample Balanced Meal Ideas for One Day

Below is an example of a full day of meals to show how balance works. Adjust portion sizes based on your age, activity level, and hunger.

1. **Breakfast**: Whole-grain toast with a small spread of peanut butter, a side of low-fat yogurt with sliced bananas, and a glass of water.

2. **Morning Snack**: Carrot sticks with hummus.

3. **Lunch**: Bean and veggie wrap using a whole wheat tortilla, black beans, chopped peppers, a little cheese or avocado, and some lettuce. Have a piece of fruit for dessert.

4. **Afternoon Snack**: A handful of nuts and a cup of herbal tea or water.

5. **Dinner**: Grilled fish (or tofu), brown rice, and steamed broccoli. For flavor, drizzle a bit of lemon juice or olive oil. Finish with mixed berries for dessert.

This plan includes whole grains, lean protein or plant-based proteins, plenty of fruits and veggies, and a moderate amount of healthy fats.

---

## Tracking Your Meals

Some people like to keep a food journal or use an app to note what they eat. This can help you see if you are missing certain foods. However, it is not necessary for everyone. If you are generally mindful about your choices and include lots of different fruits, vegetables, and protein sources, you might not need to track every bite.

---

## Cooking Methods That Support Balance

1. **Baking and Roasting**: Requires little added fat if you use non-stick trays or parchment paper. Great for vegetables, fish, or lean meats.

2. **Steaming**: Keeps nutrients in vegetables because you do not boil them away in water.

3. **Grilling**: Can give meats and vegetables a tasty flavor without too much added fat.

4. **Stir-Frying**: Quick cooking with minimal oil if you use a good pan or wok.

## Making Balanced Meals Enjoyable

Eating well does not mean giving up flavor. Here are ways to enjoy your balanced meals:

- **Use Herbs and Spices**: Basil, oregano, thyme, rosemary, cinnamon, nutmeg, ginger, garlic, and onions can make meals more exciting.

- **Try Different Cuisines**: Foods from around the world often feature lots of vegetables, beans, and whole grains in creative ways.

- **Eat Slowly and Mindfully**: Notice the colors, textures, and tastes of your food. Pause to appreciate your meal.

# CHAPTER 10

## Eating Well on a Budget

Many people worry that eating healthy foods costs too much. While some fresh items or special products can be pricey, there are plenty of ways to eat well without spending a fortune. With careful planning, smart shopping, and a little creativity, you can enjoy balanced and tasty meals while keeping an eye on your wallet. This chapter will share tips and ideas on how to stretch your money and still get the nutrients you need.

## Why Budget-Friendly Eating Matters

1. **Financial Savings**
   Spending too much on takeout or expensive grocery items can affect your financial well-being. Learning how to make the most of your food budget helps you save for other things in life.

2. **Health Benefits**
   Cheaper does not have to mean less nutritious. In fact, many budget-friendly choices—like beans, oats, eggs, and vegetables—can be packed with nutrients.

3. **Less Food Waste**
   When you plan carefully, you waste less. This not only saves money but also helps the environment by reducing the amount of food thrown away.

## Plan Before You Shop

One of the best ways to keep your food spending under control is to plan ahead.

1. **Set a Weekly Menu**

    - Look at your schedule. Decide how many meals you need to cook at home.

    - Choose recipes or meal ideas that share ingredients, so you can buy in bulk.

    - Include options you know how to cook and enjoy.

2. **Check Your Kitchen First**

    - See what foods you already have. A can of beans in the cupboard or some frozen veggies might help you skip buying extra items.

    - Make a list of what you are missing and need to buy.

3. **Create a Shopping List**

    - Write down everything you need for the planned meals.

    - Stick to your list in the store to avoid impulse buys that can raise your bill.

## Shop Smart

When you head to the store (or shop online), these steps can help you save money:

1. **Compare Prices**
Different stores sometimes sell the same items at different prices. If possible, check flyers or websites to find the best deals. You can also compare unit prices on the shelf labels to see which brand is cheaper per ounce or gram.

2. **Buy in Bulk (When It Makes Sense)**
Foods like rice, oats, beans, and lentils are often cheaper per unit when purchased in larger bags. Just make sure you have space to store them and that you will use them before they go bad.

3. **Look for Discounts and Sales**

    - Check for weekly deals. Maybe fresh produce is on sale if it is in season.

    - Look for "manager's special" items that need to be sold soon. If you can cook or freeze them right away, you can save a lot.

4. **Consider Store Brands**
Many supermarkets have their own brands for foods like cereal, bread, and canned goods. These can be cheaper than name brands and often have similar quality.

5. **Avoid Shopping While Hungry**
When you are hungry, everything looks good, and you might buy more than planned, including expensive or less healthy snacks.

# Affordable Protein Sources

Protein can sometimes be costly, but you have many budget-friendly choices if you know where to look:

1. **Beans and Lentils**

    - Often sold in dry bags or cans.

    - Dry beans cost less over time, though they take more preparation.

    - Add beans to soups, stews, salads, or mash them into spreads. They are full of protein, fiber, and minerals.

2. **Eggs**

    - Usually cheaper compared to many meats.

    - Easy to cook and can be used for breakfast, lunch, or dinner.

    - Boil a few eggs in advance and keep them in the fridge for quick meals.

3. **Canned Fish**

    - Tuna or sardines can be cheaper options than fresh fish.

    - They store well and can be added to salads, sandwiches, or mixed into pasta.

    - Look for varieties packed in water instead of oil to reduce added fat.

4. **Cheaper Cuts of Meat**

    - Chicken thighs, drumsticks, or bone-in chicken pieces are often less expensive than boneless chicken breasts.
    - Lean ground turkey or ground beef can be stretched by mixing in beans or vegetables.
    - Slow cooking tough cuts can make them tender and tasty, saving money compared to prime cuts.

5. **Tofu and Tempeh**

    - Plant-based options that can be cheaper than meats in some areas.
    - Absorb flavors from sauces or seasonings, making them versatile for stir-fries or stews.

---

## Fruits and Vegetables Without Breaking the Bank

Fruits and veggies supply vitamins, minerals, and fiber, but fresh versions can sometimes be costly, especially out of season.

1. **Buy Seasonal Produce**

    - Fruits and vegetables that are in season often cost less and taste better.
    - If you see a sale on a certain produce, build some meals around it.

2. **Frozen Options**

    - Frozen vegetables and fruits are usually picked at peak ripeness and quickly frozen, so they keep many nutrients.
    - They can be cheaper, do not spoil quickly, and you can use as much as you need at a time.

3. **Canned Vegetables and Fruits**

    - Often cheaper than fresh and can last a long time.
    - Look for low-sodium or no-salt-added vegetables.
    - Choose fruits canned in juice rather than syrup to avoid too much sugar.

4. **Buy in Bulk and Share**

    - If you find a great deal on a large bag of apples or onions, consider sharing with a friend or neighbor so nothing goes to waste.

---

## Starches and Whole Grains on a Budget

Whole grains provide long-lasting energy and extra nutrients like fiber:

1. **Oats**

    - Oatmeal is usually cheaper than many boxed cereals.

- You can use oats in baking, as a breakfast cereal, or even to thicken meatloaf or burgers.

2. **Rice**

    - Brown rice has more fiber and nutrients than white rice.

    - A large bag of rice can last a long time, especially if you store it in a sealed container.

3. **Pasta**

    - Whole wheat pasta can be low-cost.

    - You can cook a large batch and mix it with vegetables or a simple sauce.

4. **Other Grains**

    - Barley, bulgur, and corn grits can be cheaper than fancy quinoa. Check the bulk aisle if your store has one.

---

## Budget-Friendly Meal Ideas

You do not need fancy recipes to eat well on a budget. Try these simple ideas:

1. **Hearty Soup or Stew**

    - Base: Low-sodium broth or water.

- Protein: Beans, lentils, or cheaper cuts of meat.
- Veggies: Frozen or fresh carrots, onions, celery, potatoes.
- Spices: A bit of salt, pepper, herbs, or garlic.
  You can make a big pot and have leftovers. Pair it with whole grain bread if you like.

2. **Stir-Fry with Rice**

    - Protein: Tofu, eggs, or sliced chicken thighs.
    - Veggies: Frozen stir-fry mix or fresh veggies on sale.
    - Sauce: A small amount of soy sauce or a homemade sauce (water, cornstarch, a bit of low-sugar ketchup, garlic).
    - Rice: Cook brown rice in bulk and use it for several meals.

3. **Bean Burritos**

    - Beans: Black beans or pinto beans.
    - Wraps: Whole wheat tortillas (check for store brands).
    - Extras: Shredded lettuce, chopped tomatoes, a spoonful of salsa, or grated cheese.
      Beans are cost-effective, and the meal can be put together quickly.

4. **Egg-Based Meals**

    - Omelets with leftover vegetables and a little cheese.

    - Breakfast burritos with scrambled eggs and beans.

    - Frittatas with potatoes, onions, and spinach.
      Eggs can become the star of a budget-friendly dinner.

---

## Buying in Bulk and Storing Properly

Buying larger bags or containers can help you save, but only if you store them correctly so they do not spoil:

1. **Dry Goods**

    - Keep rice, beans, pasta, and oats in airtight containers in a cool, dry place.

    - Label containers with the purchase date to use older supplies first.

2. **Proteins**

    - If you buy a big package of meat, separate it into meal-size portions before freezing.

    - Canned tuna or chicken can last for a long time in the cupboard.

3. **Fruits and Vegetables**

    - Freeze extra fruits like bananas before they go bad. Use them in smoothies or baked goods.

    - Chop and freeze vegetables if you bought too many. They can go into soups or stir-fries later.

---

## Reducing Food Waste

Wasted food is wasted money. Try these tips to get the most out of what you buy:

1. **Use Leftovers Wisely**

    - If you have leftover chicken, add it to a salad or wrap the next day.

    - Leftover vegetables can go into a soup or be blended into a sauce.

    - Stale bread can become breadcrumbs or croutons.

2. **Store Produce Correctly**

    - Some veggies like carrots, celery, and lettuce stay crisp in the fridge wrapped or in sealed bags.

    - Onions and potatoes do better in a cool, dark place, but not in the fridge.

    - Apples can last longer in the fridge, while bananas are better at room temperature (until ripe).

3. **Check Dates**
    - "Sell by" or "Best by" dates do not always mean the food is spoiled right after. Use your senses (look, smell, taste a small bit) to decide if something is still good, but always be cautious with foods that spoil easily.

---

## Cooking at Home vs. Eating Out

Eating out can be fun, but it can also cost a lot. Fast food may look cheap, but the expenses can add up if you do it often. Home-cooked meals:

- Usually cost less per serving.
- Let you control ingredients like salt, sugar, and fat.
- Often leave you with leftovers you can eat later.

If you still want an occasional treat, budget for it. For instance, plan to cook at home most days and allow for one takeout meal a week.

---

## Healthy Swaps to Save Money

1. **Skip Soda, Drink Water**
   Sugary drinks can be pricey and do not help your health. Water is free or low-cost and hydrates you better.

2. **Limit Packaged Snacks**
   Chips, cookies, and candy might seem cheap, but the costs add up. Buying in bulk and portioning them out (or making homemade treats) can be cheaper.

3. **Avoid "Single-Serve" Portions**
   Items packaged in small servings often cost more per ounce. Buy larger packages and portion them yourself at home.

## Use Simple Recipes

Some fancy recipes use unusual or pricey ingredients, but simple dishes can be just as tasty:

- **Basic Tomato Sauce**: Canned tomatoes, onions, garlic, and a little oil can make a cheaper sauce than most store-bought jars.

- **Vegetable Soup**: Water, bouillon (or low-sodium broth), mixed vegetables (fresh, frozen, or canned), plus leftover meat or beans for protein.

- **Baked Chicken**: Season chicken pieces with salt, pepper, and a bit of herbs, then bake. Serve with rice and frozen vegetables for an easy meal.

## Grow Your Own (If You Can)

Some people have space for a small garden or containers on a balcony or windowsill. Herbs like basil, parsley, or chives can be grown in pots. This saves money at the store and provides fresh flavors. Some vegetables can be grown in small spaces too, like tomatoes or peppers in containers. Even if you cannot grow a lot, a few herbs can lower your grocery bill and add taste to your meals.

## Make the Most of Leftovers

Turning leftovers into new dishes can save money and keep meals interesting:

- **Leftover Rice**: Fry it with a scrambled egg, some veggies, and a drizzle of soy sauce for homemade fried rice.

- **Leftover Vegetables**: Put them in an omelet, or blend them into a soup or pasta sauce.

- **Leftover Meat**: Shred and add to tacos, quesadillas, or burritos.

- **Leftover Beans**: Mash them with spices to make a spread or add them to salads.

## Share Resources and Skills

Sometimes, you can team up with friends or neighbors to cut costs:

- **Bulk Buying**: Split big purchases of rice, beans, or other staples.

- **Group Cooking**: Cook large meals together and share the food.

- **Recipe Sharing**: Swap ideas for budget-friendly meals.

- **Potluck Meals**: Each person brings one dish, so you can enjoy a variety without buying everything yourself.

## Staying Inspired

Eating on a budget can feel challenging if you keep cooking the same things. To stay motivated:

- Look up new recipes that use low-cost ingredients you enjoy.

- Explore online videos for budget-friendly meal prep.

- Check out cookbooks at the library for fresh ideas.

- Remember that even simple changes can keep meals interesting—like adding a new spice or switching up your veggies.

---

## A Sample Budget-Friendly Meal Plan for a Day

Here is one example of how you might plan a full day of eating without spending too much:

1. **Breakfast**:

    - Oatmeal topped with banana slices and a little peanut butter.

    - Water or plain tea.
      *(Oats and bananas are affordable and filling.)*

2. **Lunch**:

    - Bean and vegetable soup (homemade with canned beans, carrots, onions, and celery).

- A piece of whole wheat bread.
  *(Soups stretch ingredients and can feed several people.)*

3. **Afternoon Snack**:

    - A hard-boiled egg and a few whole wheat crackers.
      *(Eggs are a cheap protein source.)*

4. **Dinner**:

    - Baked chicken drumsticks (cheaper cut than chicken breast), seasoned with herbs.
    - Brown rice cooked in bulk.
    - Steamed or frozen vegetables on the side.
      *(Easy to prep, and leftovers can be reused in another meal.)*

This menu uses straightforward, low-cost items that are generally available in most grocery stores.

---

## Conclusion of Chapter 10

Eating well does not have to empty your wallet. By planning ahead, shopping smart, and focusing on affordable staples like beans, eggs, and seasonal or frozen produce, you can prepare balanced meals on a tight budget. Storing food properly, using leftovers, and finding creative ways to flavor dishes also help save money and reduce waste. With these tips, you can enjoy wholesome, varied meals every day without spending more than you have. Good nutrition is possible for everyone when you use the right strategies and make the most of simple, nutrient-packed foods.

# CHAPTER 11

## Planning Your Daily Food Routine

A daily food routine is a plan for how, when, and what you eat each day. It helps you organize your meals and snacks in a way that fits your schedule and gives your body the nutrients and energy it needs. Unlike simply having random meals here and there, following a regular eating pattern can support stable energy levels, better focus, and a more comfortable relationship with food. This chapter explores how to design a flexible but consistent food routine, why timing matters, and tips to make everyday eating simpler and more nourishing.

## Why a Daily Food Routine Is Helpful

1. **Consistent Energy**
   When you eat at roughly the same times each day, your body becomes familiar with the pattern. It expects fuel at those times and learns how to use it more steadily. Random eating or skipping meals can lead to low energy or sudden cravings.

2. **Supports Healthy Habits**
   Having a routine makes it easier to include balanced foods. You can plan meals with vegetables, whole grains, and lean proteins. A set schedule also helps you avoid rushing to grab fast food or snacks without nutrients.

3. **Prevents Overeating**
   If you skip meals or wait too long to eat, you might feel very hungry and consume too much in one sitting. By spreading meals and snacks throughout the day, you are less likely to overeat later on.

4. **Reduces Stress**
   Deciding what to eat at the last minute can be stressful. A routine removes guesswork. You already know when and what you will eat, so it becomes part of your normal day.

5. **Works with Your Body's Clock**
   Your body has its own internal clock (sometimes called the circadian rhythm). Eating on a regular schedule can align with that clock, supporting good digestion and sleep patterns.

---

## Finding the Right Meal Frequency

Meal frequency is how often you eat each day. Some people do well with three main meals, while others enjoy having smaller meals plus snacks. There is no single right number—it depends on your age, activity level, and personal preferences.

1. **Three Meals a Day**

    - **Breakfast:** Helps you start the morning with energy, especially after several hours without food overnight.

    - **Lunch:** Refuels you midday to keep you going.

    - **Dinner:** An evening meal that can be a chance to gather with family or friends.

2. This classic pattern works well for many people. If you get hungry between these meals, you can add a small snack.

3. **Five or Six Smaller Meals**

    - Spreads your calorie intake throughout the day.

    - May help some people who feel shaky if they do not eat for long periods or athletes who need extra energy.

    - Requires more frequent meal prep and planning.

4. This approach can help if you prefer lighter meals but get hungry every few hours.

5. **Two or Three Meals Plus Planned Snacks**

    - Some people have a snack between breakfast and lunch, and another between lunch and dinner.

    - These snacks can be small but balanced, like yogurt with fruit, or whole-grain crackers with cheese.

6. Carefully planned snacks help prevent overeating later and keep energy stable, especially for children, teens, or those with very active schedules.

---

# Matching Your Meals to Your Day's Activities

Your daily routine probably includes work, school, sports, or hobbies. Meal planning can change based on what you do and when:

1. **Morning Activities**
    - If you have sports or a workout in the morning, you might need a bigger breakfast with carbohydrates and protein.

- If your morning is calm, a lighter breakfast could be enough, maybe a bowl of oatmeal or an egg on toast.

2. **Afternoon Tasks**

    - Lunchtime might need to be quick if you have a short break. Make sure you have something balanced and ready to go instead of skipping.

    - If you do not have an afternoon snack, you might become very hungry before dinner, so consider adding fruit with peanut butter or a handful of nuts around mid-afternoon.

3. **Evening Events**
    - If you have sports practice, music lessons, or other activities in the evening, plan an afternoon snack. Then have dinner afterward or a lighter dinner before and a small snack later.

    - If you eat dinner too late, you might struggle with digestion before bedtime. Try to finish your main meal a couple of hours before you sleep.

4. **Weekends vs. Weekdays**
    - Weekdays might be more structured: breakfast before school or work, lunch break at a set time, dinner in the evening.

    - Weekends can be more flexible. Some people sleep in and miss breakfast, then have brunch. While occasional changes are okay, try not to let your entire routine become chaotic, or it may affect your energy levels and eating patterns for the next week.

## Listening to Your Hunger and Fullness Signals

Even with a solid routine, it is important to pay attention to what your body tells you:

1. **Recognize Hunger**

    - Signals include a rumbling stomach, feeling a bit lightheaded, or low energy.

    - If you feel actual hunger, it is usually time to eat, even if it is not the exact time you planned.

2. **Feeling Full**

    - Try to stop eating when you feel comfortably satisfied, not stuffed.

    - Eating slowly can help you notice the point where you have had enough.

3. **Avoid Forced Eating**

    - If your routine says it is lunchtime but you are truly not hungry, you can have a smaller meal or wait a little.

    - However, if skipping leads you to eat too much later, try adjusting portion sizes or snack times.

## Structuring Your Day with Meals and Snacks

Here is an example of how someone might plan a day. Note that portion sizes and specific food choices will vary based on personal needs:

1. **Early Morning (6-7 AM)**

    - **Breakfast:** Whole-grain cereal with milk and sliced fruit, or eggs with whole-wheat toast. A glass of water or tea.

2. **Mid-Morning (9-10 AM)**

    - **Snack (if needed):** A small yogurt, piece of fruit, or a handful of nuts.

3. **Lunch (12-1 PM)**

    - **Main Meal:** Could be a whole-grain sandwich with lean meat or beans and lots of veggies. Or maybe leftovers from dinner. A side of fresh fruit or a small salad. Water to drink.

4. **Afternoon (3-4 PM)**
    - **Snack (optional):** Depending on hunger, this might be a piece of cheese and whole-grain crackers, sliced vegetables with hummus, or a banana with nut butter.

5. **Dinner (6-7 PM)**

    - **Main Meal:** Lean protein (chicken, fish, tofu, or beans), a whole-grain side (brown rice, quinoa, or whole-wheat pasta), and cooked or fresh vegetables. Water or milk to drink, depending on preference.

6. **Evening (8-9 PM)**

    - **Light Snack (only if really hungry):** A piece of fruit, a small mug of warm milk, or a few whole-grain crackers if dinner was early. Avoid heavy meals right before bed.

This schedule is flexible. The times and meal sizes can shift to match different lifestyles, like an earlier lunch break at school or a late evening sports practice.

---

## Meal Timing and Physical Activity

Exercise can change how you plan your meals. If you have practice or a workout:

- **Before Exercise:** Have a light snack with easy-to-digest carbs and a bit of protein about 30-60 minutes before. For example, half a peanut butter sandwich or a small bowl of oatmeal with fruit.

- **After Exercise:** Within an hour, eat a balanced meal or snack with both carbs and protein to help muscles recover—maybe a tuna sandwich or a smoothie with yogurt and fruits.

For intense or long-lasting workouts, you might need an extra snack or slightly bigger meals on those days.

---

## Breakfast: The Morning Kickstart

Breakfast wakes up your metabolism after a night without food. While some people skip it, having something in the morning can:

- Give you energy for school or work.

- Help you avoid grabbing less healthy snacks later.

- Support clear thinking and a stable mood.

If you are short on time, plan simple breakfasts like:

- Overnight oats you prepared the night before.

- A quick smoothie with milk, fruit, and a spoonful of nut butter.

- Whole-grain toast with egg or cheese.

Making breakfast ahead or choosing grab-and-go items (like fruit and a cheese stick) can help keep you on track.

---

## Lunch: Midday Fuel

Lunch refuels you and keeps you productive until later in the afternoon:

- **Pack Your Lunch:** Making your own lunch helps control portions and ingredients. You can include leftovers, sandwiches, salads, or wraps with veggies.

- **Avoid Skipping:** If you wait until mid-afternoon, you might experience a drop in energy and concentration. This can lead to overeating at dinner.

- **Add Veggies or Fruit:** If you have a sandwich, pair it with carrot sticks or a small side salad. This boosts vitamins and fiber.

## Dinner: The Day's Wind-Down

Dinner is often a time to sit down with family or friends:

- **Balance on Your Plate:** Aim for a mix of protein, healthy carbs, and vegetables.

- **Watch Out for Overeating:** Eating very large meals late at night can disrupt sleep.

- **Family Meal Benefits:** Studies show that families who eat dinner together often choose more nutritious meals and spend quality time talking about their day.

## Snack Strategies

Snacks should be planned parts of your day, not just random munching:

1. **Healthy Snack Ideas**

    - Fruit with low-fat cheese.

    - Whole-grain crackers and hummus.

    - Yogurt with a sprinkle of nuts or seeds.

- Homemade trail mix with nuts, seeds, and a small amount of dried fruit.

- Sliced veggies with guacamole or bean dip.

2. **When to Snack**

    - If you feel hungry between meals and the next meal is more than an hour away.

    - Before or after physical activities if you need extra energy.

    - During a long day at school or work, where lunch might be early and dinner is late.

3. **Portion Control**

    - Snacks can turn into full meals if portions are too big.

    - Use small containers or cups to limit mindless eating.

---

# Preparing Meals in Batches

A daily routine often works better if you have healthy foods ready to go:

1. **Cooking in Large Batches**

    - Make a big pot of soup or stew. Freeze or refrigerate in individual portions. Reheat for quick lunches or dinners.

- Bake or grill chicken breasts or tofu slices in advance to use in salads or wraps.

2. **Wash and Chop Vegetables**

    - Rinse and cut carrots, peppers, or celery in one session. Store them in the fridge for fast snacks or to add into recipes.
    - Prepare salad greens so they are ready to toss with dressing.

3. **Overnight or Slow Cooker Meals**

    - Slow cookers allow you to start a meal in the morning and have it ready by dinnertime.
    - Overnight preparations can simplify breakfast routines (like overnight oats).

---

## Flexible Approaches for Different Ages

- **Children:** May need 3 meals and 1-2 snacks due to smaller stomachs and higher nutrient demands for growth. Encourage them to listen to hunger signals but provide structured mealtimes.

- **Teens:** Often have unpredictable schedules. Sports, studying, and social events can shift mealtimes. Encourage consistent meals and healthy snacks to support growth and activity.

- **Adults:** Work schedules can shape meal timing. Planning lunches or healthy take-along snacks keeps you from relying too often on vending machines or fast food.

- **Older Adults:** Appetite might decrease, but nutrient needs remain. Smaller, more frequent meals with high-quality protein and a variety of fruits and vegetables can help.

## Handling Social Events and Special Occasions

Sometimes your routine will shift due to birthday parties, holidays, or dining out with friends. A rigid plan can create stress, so allow flexibility:

- **Adjust Around the Event:** If you know you will have a big dinner out, have a lighter lunch.

- **Focus on Balance:** At a party with desserts and snacks, choose a few treats that really appeal to you, but also include some fruits or veggies if available.

- **Return to Your Usual Routine Next Meal:** One special event will not undo your healthy habits if you go back to your normal pattern afterward.

## Staying Hydrated

Water plays a key role in any daily food routine:

- **Drink Regularly:** Have a glass of water with meals and sips in between.

- **Add Flavor:** Use fruit slices or cucumber slices if plain water gets boring.

- **Check Thirst Cues:** Thirst might sometimes feel like hunger. Drink water first to see if that solves the urge to snack.

---

## Adjusting for Busy Mornings or Evenings

If your mornings are hectic, think about ways to simplify:

- **Breakfast On-the-Go:** Prepare a smoothie the night before (blend in the morning) or grab a homemade muffin with a piece of fruit.

- **Set Out Items Ahead of Time:** Lay out cereal, bowls, or pack lunches before bed, so you are not rushing at dawn.

If your evenings are busy:

- **Use a Slow Cooker or Instant Cooker:** Meals can be ready when you arrive home.

- **Plan Quick-Cook Recipes:** Stir-fries, salads with pre-cooked protein, or simple pasta dishes can come together quickly.

---

## Dealing with Changing Schedules

Life can change—new jobs, school schedules, or family additions might shift meal times:

- **Stay Flexible:** Adjust your routine in small steps. If you move from a job starting at 9 AM to one starting at 7 AM, your breakfast might move earlier, and lunch might move earlier too.

- **Prepare for Surprises:** Keep healthy snack bars or nuts in your bag or desk for days when routines suddenly change.

- **Set Boundaries:** If your new schedule forces you to skip meals too often, think about solutions like meal prepping or packing more convenient lunches.

---

## Mindful Eating

Mindful eating means paying close attention to the foods you choose and how you feel when you eat. It can fit well into a routine:

1. **Eat Without Distractions When Possible**

    - Turning off the TV or stepping away from the computer during meals helps you focus on taste and fullness signals.

2. **Taste and Texture**

    - Notice flavors and textures. This can help you enjoy your meal more and feel satisfied.

3. **Pace**

    - Eat slowly, take small breaks, and give your body time to tell you if you are still hungry.

---

## Avoiding the "All or Nothing" Attitude

Your plan might not be perfect every day. You might oversleep and miss breakfast once, or end up with a late-night meal after a busy evening:

- **Learn from It:** If you miss lunch and end up overeating at dinner, note what happened. Next time, try packing a snack or setting a reminder.

- **Get Back on Track:** One day's slip-up does not ruin your overall routine. Focus on tomorrow and do your best to follow your plan.

- **Celebrate Little Successes:** Every balanced meal or well-planned snack is a step in the right direction.

---

## Sample Daily Routine for a Weekday

Below is an example showing how you might arrange meals around a typical schedule. Times can shift based on personal needs:

### 6:30 AM – Wake Up

- Drink a glass of water to start the day.

### 7:00 AM – Breakfast

- Whole-grain toast, scrambled eggs, and fruit.

- Cup of milk or tea.

**10:00 AM – Light Snack (If Needed)**

- Greek yogurt with a drizzle of honey or a piece of fruit.

**12:30 PM – Lunch**

- Salad with lettuce, chopped vegetables, grilled chicken, and a vinaigrette dressing.
- Whole-grain roll on the side.
- Water to drink.

**3:30 PM – Afternoon Snack**

- Slice of cheese and whole-wheat crackers.
- Another glass of water.

**6:30 PM – Dinner**

- Brown rice, steamed broccoli, salmon (or tofu), lightly seasoned.
- A piece of fruit for dessert if desired.

**8:00-9:00 PM – Relax/Light Snack (Optional)**

- If still hungry, a warm cup of milk or a small handful of nuts.
- Aim to finish eating at least an hour before bedtime.

This schedule offers structure but can be changed for earlier or later times, bigger lunches, or smaller dinners depending on your personal life.

## Using Tools to Help

- **Calendars or Apps:** Some people track meal times and food choices using a calendar, a meal-planning board, or apps that send reminders.

- **Alarm or Timer:** Setting an alarm for snack breaks can be helpful if you are busy and forget to eat, or to remind you not to delay meals too long.

- **Meal Prep Containers:** Buying or reusing containers that are portioned into sections can make it simpler to pack balanced meals.

## Conclusion of Chapter 11

A daily food routine is about finding a comfortable, repeatable pattern that meets your nutritional needs while fitting your life. There is no single right way for everyone, but the common goal is to stay consistent enough that your body receives regular fuel, nutrients, and hydration. By planning out main meals and sensible snacks, listening to your body's hunger signals, and allowing for flexibility when events change your schedule, you can build a routine that supports steady energy, better focus, and overall well-being. Whether you have three bigger meals or several smaller ones each day, the key is to maintain a pattern that is balanced, nourishing, and sustainable for you in the long run.

# CHAPTER 12

## Smart Snacking and Sweet Treats

Snacks and sweet treats can be enjoyable parts of your day, but they can also become areas where too much sugar, salt, or unhealthy fats sneak into your diet. Understanding how to choose or make snacks that help your body—and how to enjoy sweets without going overboard—can make a big difference in how you feel. This chapter will focus on smart snacking strategies, handling sweet cravings, and keeping treats in balance with the rest of your eating habits.

## Why Snacking Matters

Snacking is not just about grabbing something to munch on when you are bored. Planned, balanced snacks can:

- **Fill Nutrient Gaps**: If your main meals miss certain nutrients, a healthy snack can help make up for it.

- **Steady Energy**: Instead of feeling a big drop in energy between meals, a well-chosen snack can keep you going.

- **Prevent Overeating Later**: If you get too hungry, you might eat more than you need at your next meal. Snacks can keep hunger in check.

However, snacking can turn into a problem if snacks are always high in sugar, salt, or fat, or if you snack out of boredom rather than true hunger.

# Choosing Better Snacks

1. **Protein + Fiber**

   - Combining protein and fiber helps you feel satisfied longer. Examples: Greek yogurt with berries, cheese sticks with whole-grain crackers, or a small handful of nuts and fruit.

2. **Whole, Natural Foods**

   - Fresh fruits, vegetables, nuts, seeds, and plain yogurt are less processed, so they often contain more nutrients and less added sugar or salt.

3. **Watch Portion Sizes**

   - Even healthy foods can lead to weight gain if eaten in big amounts. Using smaller bowls or pre-portioned containers can help.

4. **Avoid Mindless Snacking**

   - Eating in front of a screen can cause you to lose track of how much you have eaten. If possible, have your snack on a plate or in a small bowl, and step away from distractions for a few minutes.

## Healthy Snack Ideas for Different Times of Day

- **Morning Snack**:
  If you had an early breakfast, you might need a snack around mid-morning. Good options include a small banana with peanut butter, carrot sticks with hummus, or a hard-boiled egg and a piece of fruit.

- **Afternoon Snack**:
  After school or during a break from work, choose something to keep you going until dinner. Try air-popped popcorn sprinkled with a little seasoning (not too much salt), a slice of whole-grain bread with mashed avocado, or a small container of cottage cheese with diced pineapple.

- **Evening Snack**:
  Sometimes dinner is early, or you feel a bit of hunger before bed. A light snack like half a cup of oatmeal with berries, a glass of low-fat milk, or a few whole-grain crackers and cheese can work. Avoid large or heavy snacks right before bedtime, which may disrupt sleep.

---

## Tips for Managing Sweet Cravings

It is natural to want sweet flavors sometimes. But sugary snacks and desserts can add extra calories without many nutrients. How can you satisfy a sweet tooth in a healthier way?

1. **Choose Fruits**

    - Many fruits are sweet and also give vitamins, minerals, and fiber. Berries, grapes, or melon chunks can be a refreshing treat.

- If you freeze grapes or banana slices, they taste even sweeter and can mimic dessert-like textures.

2. **Dark Chocolate**

    - A small square of dark chocolate (with a high cocoa percentage) can be a treat. It often has less sugar than milk chocolate.

    - Enjoy it slowly, letting each piece melt in your mouth, rather than eating a large candy bar all at once.

3. **Pair Sweets with Healthier Foods**

    - Dip strawberries in a bit of melted dark chocolate instead of eating a whole chocolate bar.

    - Top plain yogurt with a small drizzle of honey or fruit jam, rather than buying heavily sweetened yogurts.

4. **Limit Portion Sizes**

    - If you love ice cream, consider having a small scoop instead of a large bowl.

    - You can also choose sorbet or frozen yogurt if you prefer. Check labels for sugar content, though, because some frozen yogurts can still be high in sugar.

5. **Homemade Desserts**

    - Baking at home allows you to control how much sugar you use.

- You can try recipes that reduce sugar or use natural sweeteners like applesauce or mashed bananas.

## Balance Treats within Your Routine

Having a plan for when and how to enjoy sweet treats can keep them from becoming too frequent:

- **Designated Dessert Time**: Maybe your family decides on desserts after dinner a few nights a week, not every day.

- **Skip Sugary Beverages**: Instead of soda or sweet tea, drink water or unsweetened beverages, and save your sugar "allowance" for a dessert you truly enjoy.

- **Occasional Treats**: Save sugary treats for special occasions or weekends, so they remain something fun rather than a daily habit.

## Making Store-Bought Snacks Smarter

When you buy snacks at the store, it can be easy to get lost in bright packages. Here is how to pick more wisely:

1. **Read Labels for Added Sugars and Sodium**

    - Check the ingredient list and nutrition facts. Some items might look healthy but hide a lot of sugar or salt.

    - Keep an eye on portion sizes. A bag might say "100 calories per serving," but one bag can have multiple servings.

2. **Look for Whole Grains**

    - Choose whole-grain crackers or granola bars with oats, brown rice, or whole wheat as the first ingredient.

    - Avoid those loaded with icing or candy bits.

3. **Pick Lower-Sugar Options**

    - Yogurts can be healthy, but some have as much sugar as desserts. Look for plain or low-sugar versions, then add your own fruit.

4. **Be Wary of Fat-Free Claims**

    - Many "fat-free" or "low-fat" snacks compensate by adding more sugar or salt to maintain flavor. Check the nutrition label to see what is really in it.

---

## Savory Snacks: Going Beyond Chips

Sometimes we crave a salty or crunchy snack. Instead of reaching for potato chips:

- **Air-Popped Popcorn**: A whole grain, high-fiber snack. Season lightly with herbs, or just a little salt.

- **Whole-Grain Crackers**: Pair with salsa, hummus, or a bean dip.

- **Roasted Chickpeas**: Crunchy, savory, and full of protein. You can roast them at home with a bit of oil and spices.

- **Baked Veggie Chips**: Sweet potato chips or kale chips can be made at home. Store-bought versions might still have lots of oil or salt, so read labels carefully.

## Finding Balance for Kids and Teens

Children often reach for sweets or chips when they want a snack. Guide them toward smarter choices:

- **Make Healthy Snacks Visible**: Keep fruit in a bowl on the counter or washed and cut in the fridge. If they see it, they are more likely to pick it.

- **Limit Sugary Treats at Home**: If cookies or candy are not there, kids cannot grab them as easily. Instead, stock up on flavored rice cakes, yogurt tubes (low-sugar), or fruit cups in 100% juice.

- **Set an Example**: Children learn from watching adults. If grown-ups reach for an apple with peanut butter, kids might be more open to trying it too.

## Homemade Snack Prep

Preparing snacks at home in advance can help you avoid less nutritious convenience items:

1. **Snack Boxes**

    - Use small containers with compartments for different foods: cut-up veggies, cheese cubes, grapes, and whole-grain crackers.

    - Prep these on Sunday night and store them for a couple of days.

2. **Energy Bites**

    - Mix oats, peanut butter, a little honey, and seeds into small rolled balls.

    - Keep them in the fridge for quick pick-me-ups throughout the week.

3. **Veggie Dips and Salsas**

    - Blend cooked beans or chickpeas with herbs and lemon juice to create a simple dip.

    - Prepare homemade salsa with fresh tomatoes, onions, and peppers. Use it with baked tortilla chips or veggie sticks.

---

## Timing Your Snacks

While snacking can be helpful, snacking too often might interfere with normal hunger signals or lead to overeating:

- **Plan Snack Times**: For instance, one mid-morning snack and one mid-afternoon snack if you tend to get hungry.

- **Skip "Grazing" All Day**: Constantly nibbling can make it hard to know when you are truly hungry.

- **Nighttime Snacking**: If you find yourself snacking late at night out of habit, try a bedtime routine that does not involve food, like reading a book or drinking a decaf tea.

---

## Being Mindful with Treats

1. **Enjoy the Experience**

   - If you decide to have a piece of cake or cookie, savor the taste. Eat slowly and notice the texture.

   - This can make a small portion feel more satisfying than rushing through a big slice.

2. **Share Desserts**

   - If a dessert is large, split it with a friend or family member. This way, you still get the treat but in a smaller portion.

3. **Do Not Label Treats as "Bad"**

   - Thinking of foods as "bad" can create guilt. It is okay to enjoy treats sometimes. Focus on moderation and balance the rest of your meals with nutrient-rich foods.

## Practical Ways to Reduce Sugar and Salt

1. **Flavor with Spices**

    - Cinnamon, nutmeg, or vanilla can add sweetness to oatmeal or baked goods with less sugar.

    - Herbs like basil, oregano, or thyme can boost flavor in savory snacks without too much salt.

2. **Rinse Canned Foods**

    - If you use canned beans or vegetables, rinsing them under water helps remove excess salt.

3. **Choose Fresh or Frozen Fruit**

    - Fruit canned in syrup can pack extra sugar. Pick fruit in 100% juice or water, or go for fresh or frozen options.

---

## Balancing Snacks with Main Meals

If you plan your main meals to include a balance of protein, whole grains, and vegetables, your snacks can serve as small tune-ups:

- **Add Missing Nutrients**: If your lunch lacked vegetables, choose a veggie snack in the afternoon. If you did not have enough protein at breakfast, have a protein-rich snack.

- **Mind the Overall Calories**: Snacks should not add too many calories on top of main meals. Keep them moderate in size.

- **Stay Aware of Beverages**: Sugary coffee drinks or fruit juices can sneak in extra calories. If you want something sweet to drink, try blending a small fruit smoothie with plain yogurt.

## Handling Cravings During Stress or Boredom

Sometimes we snack because we feel stressed, sad, or bored, not truly hungry:

- **Pause and Ask**: "Am I really hungry, or am I just looking for something to do?"

- **Find Another Activity**: If boredom is the issue, try a brief walk, read a book, or call a friend.

- **Healthy Stress Relief**: If stress drives snacking, consider activities like deep breathing, stretching, or writing in a journal.

## Special Events and Holidays

Celebrations often involve treats and snacks:

- **Enjoy Favorites Mindfully**: It is okay to have that holiday cookie or slice of birthday cake. Just be mindful of how many.

- **Bring a Healthy Option**: If you go to a gathering, offer to bring a fruit platter or veggie dish. That way, you know there is at least one nutritious choice.

- **Shift the Focus**: Celebrations can be about people, games, or music rather than just the food.

## Snacks for Active People

If you do sports or workouts, snacks become even more important:

- **Before Exercise**: Choose quick carbs, like a banana or half a peanut butter sandwich.

- **After Exercise**: Pair carbs with protein, such as chocolate milk, a Greek yogurt with fruit, or a turkey sandwich. This helps muscles recover.

---

## Kid-Friendly Sweet Options

For children who love sweets, you can create fun but healthier desserts:

1. **Banana "Ice Cream"**

    - Freeze bananas and then blend them until smooth. Add a spoonful of peanut butter or cocoa powder for flavor.

2. **Fruit Kabobs**

    - Thread chunks of pineapple, grapes, berries, or melon onto skewers. Dip in low-sugar yogurt.

3. **Apple Nachos**

    - Slice apples thin, drizzle with melted nut butter, and sprinkle with granola or chopped nuts.

---

## Adjusting Sweetness in Recipes

- **Reduce Sugar Gradually**: If a recipe calls for 1 cup of sugar, try 3/4 cup. Often, you will not notice a big difference.

- **Use Applesauce or Mashed Fruit**: In baked goods, replacing some sugar or butter with applesauce or pureed fruit can lower the sugar and fat content.

- **Taste Test**: If the recipe seems too mild, add a small extra spoon of sugar. This approach is still usually less than the recipe's original amount.

---

## Putting It All Together

Snacks and treats can fit into a healthy lifestyle when chosen thoughtfully. Here is how you can combine these ideas:

1. **Plan Snack Times**

    - Set one or two snack times. Have balanced mini-meals with protein, fiber, and a little healthy fat.

2. **Pick Nutritious Options**

    - Focus on fruits, vegetables, whole grains, low-fat dairy, and lean proteins.

3. **Keep Portions in Check**

    - Use smaller bowls or measure portions if you find yourself eating until a bag is empty.

4. **Enjoy Sweet Treats in Moderation**

    - Use fruit as a natural sweet source. When you want desserts, keep servings moderate and savor them slowly.

5. **Stay Hydrated**

    - Sometimes you feel hungry, but you actually need fluids. Drink water regularly.

---

## Sample Snack Schedule in a Day

Below is an example of how snacks and sweet treats might fit into a balanced day:

- **Breakfast (7:00 AM)**: Whole-grain cereal with milk, a sliced banana on top.

- **Morning Snack (10:00 AM)**: Yogurt (low sugar) with fresh berries.

- **Lunch (12:30 PM)**: Veggie wrap with beans, lettuce, tomatoes, and a side of baby carrots.

- **Afternoon Snack (3:30 PM)**: Apple slices with a tablespoon of peanut butter.

- **Dinner (6:30 PM)**: Baked chicken, brown rice, roasted vegetables.

- **Sweet Treat (7:30 PM)**: A small square of dark chocolate or homemade fruit sorbet.

- **Optional Late Snack (9:00 PM)**: Only if genuinely hungry—a small mug of warm milk or half a cup of cottage cheese with peaches.

By planning sweet treats in the evening (but in a modest portion), you satisfy your sweet tooth without constantly grazing on sugar all day.

---

## Conclusion of Chapter 12

Smart snacking and moderate sweet treats can be part of a balanced eating plan that supports overall health. Snacks serve as mini-meals, supplying nutrients and steady energy between main meals. Sweet treats, when chosen with care and eaten in modest amounts, can bring pleasure without derailing your daily routine. Whether you favor savory snacks or have a sweet tooth, learning to pick nutrient-rich options, watch portion sizes, and maintain balance helps you enjoy these foods in a way that benefits both your taste buds and your body. By planning snacks thoughtfully and savoring sweets in moderation, you can keep your eating habits on track and still enjoy the flavors you love.

---

# CHAPTER 13

## Muscle Gain through Healthy Eating

Building muscle is not only for bodybuilders or athletes. Many people want to become stronger, improve their endurance, and feel confident about how their body moves. Healthy eating is a key part of this process, because the foods you choose can either help or slow down muscle growth. This chapter will explain how the right balance of nutrients, meal timing, and practical strategies can guide your body toward steady muscle gains.

## Why Muscle Growth Matters

1. **Strength and Stability**
   Having strong muscles helps you move confidently. Day-to-day tasks like lifting groceries, playing sports, or picking up children become easier. Good muscle strength can also lower the chance of injuries.

2. **Better Body Composition**
   Muscle tissue uses energy, even when you are not moving around. If you have more muscle and a balanced approach to eating, you might maintain a healthier body shape over time.

3. **Support for Physical Activities**
   If you like basketball, dancing, running, or other sports, stronger muscles help you perform better and feel less tired afterward.

4. **Long-Term Health**
   As you age, muscle loss can occur. Working on muscle growth earlier can help slow that process and keep you active later in life.

## Basic Factors That Influence Muscle Gain

1. **Resistance Exercise**
   Activities like weightlifting, bodyweight exercises (push-ups, squats), or using resistance bands are needed to stress your muscles so they adapt and grow. The food you eat then provides the building blocks to fix and increase muscle fibers.

2. **Sufficient Calories**
   If you regularly eat fewer calories than your body uses, it is tough to add muscle. Your body needs extra energy to build and maintain muscle tissue.

3. **Proper Protein Intake**
   Protein delivers the amino acids that form new muscle fibers. While more protein does not always mean more muscle, you do need enough daily to support growth.

4. **Recovery and Rest**
   Muscles do not grow while you are actively training—they fix and develop during rest. Good sleep and rest days, combined with nutrient-rich meals, help muscles recover.

# Role of Protein in Muscle Growth

Protein is the nutrient that is often discussed the most when it comes to muscle. But how much do you really need?

1. **General Guidelines**
   Many active adults might aim for around 1.2 to 2.0 grams of protein per kilogram of body weight each day if they are trying to build muscle. For instance, a 68 kg person might need somewhere between 82 to 136 grams of protein per day. However, exact needs vary by person, level of exercise, and goals.

2. **High-Quality Protein Sources**

   - **Animal-Based**: Chicken, turkey, lean beef, fish, eggs, and low-fat dairy products. These contain a wide range of essential amino acids.

   - **Plant-Based**: Beans, lentils, tofu, tempeh, quinoa, nuts, and seeds. Combining these throughout the day can ensure you get all the important amino acids.

3. **Protein Distribution**
   Spreading your protein intake throughout the day might help your muscles use it more effectively. Instead of eating a giant steak at dinner only, include some protein at breakfast, lunch, and snacks as well.

4. **Protein Supplements**
   Some people use protein powders or shakes for convenience. This can be useful if you struggle to get enough protein through meals. Still, whole foods also provide vitamins, minerals, and fiber, so powders should not completely replace balanced meals.

## Carbohydrates for Muscle Fuel

While protein is vital, carbohydrates also matter:

1. **Energy for Workouts**
   Muscles use carbs as a primary fuel, especially in higher-intensity exercise. If you do not eat enough carbs, you might feel tired and unable to push your workouts enough to stimulate muscle growth.

2. **Replenish Glycogen**
   Glycogen is stored in your muscles and liver. After exercise, replenishing glycogen with carbs helps you recover for the next workout. Whole grains, fruits, and starchy vegetables are good choices.

3. **Balancing Carbs**
   Opt for complex carbs like brown rice, oatmeal, whole wheat bread, or quinoa. These contain fiber and release energy more steadily than sugary snacks. Fruits and dairy also offer carbs but watch out for added sugar in some products.

---

## Importance of Healthy Fats

Fats help absorb vitamins, support hormone production, and deliver lasting energy. Hormones like testosterone are linked to muscle building, so stable hormone levels are important:

1. **Healthy Fat Choices**

   - **Unsaturated Fats**: Found in avocados, nuts, seeds, and certain oils (olive, canola).

- **Omega-3 Fatty Acids**: Found in fatty fish (salmon, sardines) and in smaller amounts in walnuts and flaxseeds.

2. **Moderation**

   Fat contains more calories per gram than protein or carbs. While you need some dietary fat, going overboard can lead to extra weight that is not muscle. Focus on balanced meals instead of very high-fat diets if your goal is muscle gain without too much additional body fat.

---

## Timing Meals and Snacks for Muscle Growth

1. **Pre-Workout**

   - Eat a small meal or snack with carbs and a bit of protein about 1-2 hours before exercise.
   - Examples: Whole-grain toast with peanut butter, banana with yogurt, or oatmeal with fruit.
   - This gives you energy to train effectively.

2. **Post-Workout Window**

   - Within an hour after training, you can eat carbs and protein to help muscles recover.
   - Examples: Chocolate milk, a sandwich with lean protein, or a protein shake with fruit.

3. **Spreading Nutrients**

    - Aim for balanced meals throughout the day, not just a single high-protein meal at dinner.
    
    - Consider adding a small protein-rich snack before bed if you finish your day's meals early. This can help muscles repair during sleep.

---

## Creating a Muscle-Building Meal Plan (Example)

Here is a sample day to show how you might balance meals for muscle growth. Adjust portion sizes to match your caloric needs:

- **Breakfast (7:00 AM)**

    - Scrambled eggs (2 or 3)
    
    - Whole-grain toast with a little avocado
    
    - Mixed berries or a piece of fruit
    
    - Water

- **Mid-Morning Snack (10:00 AM)**

    - Greek yogurt with honey or sliced strawberries
    
    - Water

- **Lunch (12:30 PM)**
    - Grilled chicken breast (or tofu if plant-based)
    - Brown rice or quinoa
    - Steamed vegetables (broccoli, carrots)
    - Water or milk (if desired)
- **Pre-Workout Snack (3:30 PM)**
    - Small bowl of oatmeal with a spoonful of peanut butter
    - Water
- **Workout (4:30-5:30 PM)**
    - Stay hydrated during exercise
- **Post-Workout (6:00 PM)**
    - A fruit smoothie with a protein source (whey, soy, or pea protein) and a handful of spinach for extra nutrients
- **Dinner (7:30 PM)**
    - Salmon fillet (or tempeh if plant-based)
    - Sweet potato (baked)

- Side salad with olive oil and vinegar dressing

- Water

- **Evening Snack (9:30 PM, optional)**

    - Cottage cheese (low-fat) or a cup of low-sugar Greek yogurt

    - A few whole-grain crackers

This plan offers multiple protein sources, complex carbs, healthy fats, and spread-out meals to help muscles grow steadily.

---

## Vegetarians or Vegans Aiming for Muscle Gain

Building muscle without meat is entirely possible, but planning is key:

1. **Protein-Rich Plant Foods**

    - Beans, lentils, chickpeas, tofu, tempeh, seitan, nuts, seeds, quinoa, and soy-based products.

    - Consider combining legumes (beans, lentils) with grains (rice, wheat) to get a full range of amino acids throughout the day.

2. **Watch for Nutrient Shortfalls**

    - Iron, zinc, vitamin B12, and vitamin D might be harder to obtain if you cut out animal products. Use fortified foods or, in some cases, supplements if needed.

3. **Use Variety**

    - Mixing different plant proteins helps ensure your muscles get the amino acids they need.

    - Include protein in every meal: for example, tofu at lunch, lentil soup at dinner, a peanut butter sandwich as a snack.

---

## Hydration and Electrolytes

When you exercise, you sweat and lose fluid, along with some electrolytes like sodium and potassium:

1. **Water First**

    - Most of the time, plain water meets your hydration needs unless you do very intense or long workouts.

2. **Electrolyte Drinks**

    - Sports drinks or homemade electrolyte solutions can help if you sweat a lot or exercise more than an hour intensely.

    - Watch out for high sugar in some commercial sports drinks.

---

# Avoiding Too Much Extra Fat Gain

Some people eat large amounts of calories to gain muscle quickly, but that can also add more body fat. A balanced approach can help:

1. **Moderate Caloric Surplus**

    - Eat slightly more calories than you burn, not thousands extra. You can track your daily calorie needs based on weight, activity, and goals.

    - A small surplus of 200-300 calories per day is often enough for steady muscle gain without excessive fat gain.

2. **Protein, Not Just Junk Food**

    - Adding calories from sugary treats or fried foods will not help muscle growth as much as balanced meals.

    - Focus on nutrient-rich sources: lean meats, beans, whole grains, nuts, seeds, and healthy oils.

3. **Monitor Progress**

    - Keep an eye on how your body feels, how your workouts are going, and how clothes fit. If you are gaining too much body fat, slightly reduce your extra calories. If you are not gaining muscle, check if you need a bit more protein or total calories.

## Common Myths About Muscle Building and Food

1. **Myth**: "Only protein matters for muscle gain."
   **Truth**: While protein is vital, you also need enough carbs, healthy fats, vitamins, and minerals. A balanced diet is best.

2. **Myth**: "You have to eat meat for muscle growth."
   **Truth**: Plant-based diets can work too, as long as you get enough protein from sources like beans, lentils, tofu, and nuts.

3. **Myth**: "If you are not drinking protein shakes after every workout, you will not build muscle."
   **Truth**: Shakes are convenient, but real food can also give you the protein you need. Many people build muscle just fine through balanced meals.

4. **Myth**: "Huge amounts of protein will automatically create more muscle."
   **Truth**: Past a certain point, extra protein does not produce more muscle; it can become extra calories stored as fat. The right amount of protein, plus exercise, is what matters.

---

## Vitamins, Minerals, and Muscle Building

Your body uses a variety of vitamins and minerals to fix and grow muscle tissues. For example:

1. **Calcium**

   - Helps muscle contractions and supports bones. Found in dairy products and leafy greens.

2. **Iron**

    - Transports oxygen to muscles. Found in lean meats, beans, and fortified cereals.

3. **Magnesium**

    - Involved in muscle function and energy production. Found in nuts, seeds, and dark leafy greens.

4. **B Vitamins**

    - Help your body turn food into energy. Found in whole grains, meats, beans, and dairy.

A varied diet filled with whole grains, vegetables, fruits, lean proteins, and healthy fats usually supplies enough micronutrients. If you suspect you are low on any nutrient, you might talk with a health professional about testing or possible supplements.

---

## Avoiding Overtraining and Undereating

Sometimes people push too hard, exercising intensely without giving their body the calories or rest it needs. This can lead to burnout or even muscle loss:

1. **Signs You Might Be Overtraining**

    - Constant fatigue, poor performance in workouts, trouble sleeping, frequent illnesses, or lingering muscle soreness.

2. **Recovery Days**

    - Rest days or lighter activity days give muscles time to adapt. Gentle stretching, short walks, or easy activities keep you moving without stressing muscles too much.

3. **Balance Your Meals**

    - Skipping meals or cutting calories too low can cause your body to break down muscle for energy. Make sure you have enough fuel for your activity level.

---

# Practical Tips for Muscle-Focused Eating

1. **Meal Prep**

    - Cooking in batches lets you have protein and healthy carbs ready. For example, grill several chicken breasts or bake a big tray of tofu on Sunday, then refrigerate for the week.

    - Cook a large pot of brown rice or quinoa to pair with meals.

2. **Portable Snacks**

    - Keep protein bars (watch sugar content), small bags of nuts, or low-fat cheese sticks handy. That way, you do not skip meals if you are busy.

    - Hard-boiled eggs are also easy to take along.

3. **Easy Add-Ons**

    o   Add chickpeas or beans to salads for extra protein.

    o   Stir a spoonful of peanut butter into oatmeal.

    o   Sprinkle seeds or chopped nuts on yogurt, cereal, or pasta dishes.

4. **Focus on Foods You Enjoy**

    o   You do not have to force yourself to eat foods you dislike. There are many protein sources and healthy carbs out there. Pick ones that taste good to you, so you stick with it.

---

## Tracking Progress Wisely

While the scale can show weight changes, it does not tell you if you are gaining muscle or fat. Other ways to track progress:

1. **Performance**

    o   Keep track of your reps, sets, or workout times. If you are lifting heavier or doing more reps with ease, you are likely getting stronger.

2. **Measurements**

    o   Some people measure their arms, legs, waist, or hips. Increases in some areas (like arms) can suggest muscle growth, while changes in waist size might reflect fat changes.

3. **Visual and Feel**

    o Notice how your clothes fit or how you look in the mirror. Do you see more definition? Do you feel firmer in certain areas?

4. **Energy and Mood**

    o Muscle building should not leave you exhausted all the time. If you are eating well and balancing rest, you might feel more energetic overall.

## Addressing Underlying Health Concerns

If you find it very hard to gain muscle even with good eating and exercise:

- **Medical Check-Up**: Sometimes issues like hormone imbalances, metabolic conditions, or nutrient absorption problems can hinder progress.

- **Professional Guidance**: A dietitian or nutritionist can help you review your meal plan. A fitness trainer can check your workout program for effectiveness.

## Muscle Gain and Age Groups

1. **Teens**

    o Often gain muscle more easily because of natural growth hormones. Still, they need balanced diets that support both overall growth and muscle building.

- Avoid extremes like very high-protein diets or very low-calorie diets that can hamper growth.

2. **Adults**

    - Adults may not build muscle as quickly as teens, but it is still very possible with consistent exercise and good nutrition.
    - Busy schedules can mean meal prep is helpful to avoid missing meals.

3. **Older Adults**

    - Muscle tends to shrink with age (sarcopenia), so muscle-building nutrition and gentle resistance exercises are important.
    - Protein needs might be slightly higher, and vitamin D and calcium become more critical for bone health.

---

## Staying Motivated

Muscle growth takes time. It can be tempting to look for shortcuts or get discouraged if results do not show up right away:

1. **Set Realistic Goals**

    - Aim for steady progress, not massive changes overnight. Even small improvements in your workouts or physical changes are wins.

2. **Enjoy the Process**

    - Experiment with new recipes for your protein and carb sources.

    - Vary your workouts so you do not get bored.

3. **Celebrate Milestones**

    - When you hit a personal best at the gym or notice a positive change in the mirror, pat yourself on the back.

    - This builds confidence and keeps you going.

---

## Conclusion of Chapter 13

Muscle gain through healthy eating is about giving your body the nutrients it needs to develop stronger tissues and adapt to resistance exercise. By combining adequate protein, balanced carbs, healthy fats, and key vitamins and minerals—along with rest and smart workouts—you can see steady progress. Meal timing, portion control, and consistency are all important, but it also comes down to enjoying the foods you choose and listening to your body's signals. Muscle growth is a gradual journey, but the rewards include improved strength, better physical performance, and a healthier body for the long run.

# CHAPTER 14

## Supporting Weight Control

Maintaining a healthy weight can bring many benefits, such as steady energy, lower stress on joints, and reduced risks of certain illnesses. But "weight control" is not about extreme dieting or punishing workouts. Instead, it involves balanced eating, staying active, and paying attention to your body's signals of hunger and fullness. In this chapter, we will discuss sensible strategies for reaching or maintaining a weight that supports a strong and healthy life.

## Why a Healthy Weight Matters

1. **Overall Wellness**
   Carrying too much or too little weight can put strain on your heart, joints, and even your mental well-being. A suitable weight for your height and body type helps everything from blood pressure to mood.

2. **Energy and Stamina**
   When your weight is well-managed, everyday tasks and fun activities feel easier. You might find it less tiring to climb stairs or play sports.

3. **Long-Term Health**
   Balancing your weight can help lower the chance of developing certain health problems linked to too much body fat or, on the other hand, being underweight.

4. **Confidence and Self-Image**
   While looks are not the only factor, many people feel better about themselves when they are at a weight that feels comfortable and aligns with healthy markers.

---

## Understanding Calories and Weight

Weight change generally relates to how many calories you take in through eating versus how many your body uses:

1. **Calories In vs. Calories Out**
   - If you consume more calories than you burn, the excess may be stored as fat.
   - If you use more calories than you eat, you might lose weight.

2. **Metabolism**
   - Everyone's body uses energy at a slightly different pace. Factors like age, muscle mass, and genetic background play a role.
   - Having more muscle can raise your resting metabolism a bit because muscle tissue uses more calories than fat tissue, even at rest.

3. **Quality Over Strict Numbers**
   - While the concept of "calories in, calories out" helps, the kind of calories also matters. Eating 500 calories of sugary snacks is not the same as 500 calories of balanced proteins, carbs, and fats in terms of how you feel and how your body works.

## Finding a Balanced Approach to Weight Control

1. **Avoid Crash Diets**
   Very low-calorie diets might show quick weight loss on the scale, but often that includes losing muscle and water. Once the diet ends, old habits can lead to regaining the lost weight.

2. **Steady, Gradual Changes**
   Most guidelines suggest aiming for about 0.5 to 1 kg (1 to 2 pounds) of weight loss per week if that is your goal. If you want to gain weight healthily, a slow, steady approach is also best.

3. **Lifestyle Over Short-Term Fixes**
   Fad diets may promise dramatic results, but real success often comes from changing daily habits, like cooking healthier meals, moving more each day, and controlling portion sizes.

---

## Building an Eating Plan for Weight Control

1. **Focus on Nutrient Density**

    - Foods high in nutrients but moderate in calories include vegetables, fruits, whole grains, lean proteins, and low-fat dairy.

    - These keep you satisfied and supply your body with vitamins and minerals.

2. **Balanced Meals**

    - A good mix of protein, carbs, and healthy fats helps keep blood sugar stable.

    - Protein supports muscle, carbs give energy, and fats help with satiety (fullness).

3. **Portion Awareness**

    - Even healthy foods can lead to weight gain if eaten in very large amounts.

    - Use your plate as a guide: half for vegetables/fruits, one quarter for protein, one quarter for whole grains or starchy vegetables.

4. **Limit Added Sugars and Saturated Fats**

    - Treats like candy, soda, or fried foods can quickly exceed your calorie needs without giving much nutrition.

    - Swap them for lower-sugar, lower-fat options or enjoy them only sometimes and in small servings.

---

# Practical Weight Control Tips

1. **Start the Day with a Good Breakfast**

    - Having balanced, moderate meals from the morning on helps you avoid extreme hunger that might cause overeating later.

- For instance, a bowl of oatmeal with fruit and a side of eggs can keep you full until lunch.

2. **Snack Wisely**

    - If you like snacking, choose nutrient-rich foods: yogurt, nuts, fruits, or veggies with hummus.

    - Avoid snacking out of boredom or emotions. Ask yourself if you are truly hungry before grabbing something.

3. **Track Eating Habits (If Helpful)**

    - Writing down what you eat or using an app can reveal patterns, such as snacking too much at night or going long periods without a meal.

    - Awareness often leads to small adjustments that help you reach your goals.

4. **Watch Liquid Calories**

    - Sodas, fruit juices, and specialty coffees can contain more sugar and calories than you realize. Water or unsweetened tea/coffee are often better choices.

## Staying Active

1. **Physical Activity and Weight**

   - Exercise burns calories, but it also helps keep your muscles strong, boosts mood, and can increase your metabolic rate slightly over time by building muscle.

   - Combine aerobic activities (like walking, running, dancing) with strength exercises (like lifting weights or bodyweight exercises).

2. **Daily Movement**

   - Even small actions like taking the stairs, doing short walks, or stretching throughout the day help. You do not have to rely only on formal workouts.

3. **Make It Enjoyable**

   - Pick activities you find fun—dancing, biking, playing sports, or group classes. That way you are more likely to keep doing them.

---

## Handling Emotional Eating

Emotions can cause people to eat more or less than they need:

1. **Stress or Sadness**

   - Some people turn to comfort foods that are high in sugar or fat during hard times.

- Recognize emotional triggers. If you notice you are reaching for snacks when upset, try alternate coping skills (like a short walk, talking to a friend, or writing in a journal).

2. **Mindful Eating**

    - Eating slowly and without distractions can help you notice if you are truly hungry or just eating because of feelings.

    - Focus on the taste, texture, and smell of your food.

3. **Seek Support if Needed**

    - If emotional eating becomes a regular challenge, speaking with a counselor or mental health professional might help you address underlying reasons.

---

## Social and Cultural Factors

Weight control can be shaped by culture, family habits, or social events:

1. **Family Meals**

    - If your family often serves large portions or very rich foods, you can suggest adding more vegetables or switching to healthier cooking methods.

2. **Parties and Celebrations**

    - Social gatherings can have lots of treats. It is fine to taste them, but you can limit portions or focus on leaner options (like grilled meats instead of fried, fruit instead of cake).

3. **Peer Pressure**

    - Friends might push you to eat or drink more than you want. Practice polite ways to decline or share a smaller portion.

---

## Safe Ways to Lose Weight if Needed

If your doctor or a health professional has advised you to lose weight, keep these tips in mind:

1. **Set Realistic Targets**

    - Aim for small milestones, like losing 2-3 kg in a month, rather than huge drops right away.

    - Celebrate each step forward.

2. **Balanced Caloric Deficit**

    - Lower your daily calories slightly below what you burn.

- You can do this by eating smaller portions, choosing foods with fewer calories, and adding more exercise.

3. **Keep Protein Adequate**

    - While cutting calories, make sure you still get enough protein to protect muscle.

    - Beans, lean meats, eggs, and low-fat dairy can help.

4. **Be Patient**

    - Healthy weight loss is not a race. Quick fixes can lead to temporary results or health problems.

---

## Gaining Weight in a Healthy Way

Some people struggle with being underweight or want to gain weight for sports, muscle, or general health:

1. **Eat More Often**

    - Spread out meals and snacks to consume extra calories more comfortably.

    - Smoothies, peanut butter on whole-grain toast, and pasta with beans can add healthy calories.

2. **Nutrient-Dense Foods**

    - Avocados, nuts, seeds, and dairy products (if tolerated) are good for extra energy and nutrients.

- Avoid relying on junk food, because it might not supply enough vitamins or protein.

3. **Build Muscle**

    - Combine a higher-calorie diet with strength training to help the extra calories go toward muscle rather than just body fat.

---

## Checking Progress Beyond the Scale

1. **Measurements**

    - Keep track of your waist, hip, or arm measurements to see changes in body composition.
    - Sometimes you can be losing fat and gaining muscle, which might not show up as much on the scale.

2. **How Clothes Fit**

    - If you notice a looser or tighter fit in your clothes, that might indicate changes in body size, even if the scale number has not moved much.

3. **Energy Levels**

    - Improved energy, better workouts, or easier daily tasks can signal progress in health, even if the scale does not reflect a big shift.

## Common Pitfalls and How to Avoid Them

1. **Yo-Yo Dieting**

    - Rapidly changing from one diet to another can disrupt your metabolism and lead to weight regain. Focus on steady, permanent changes.

2. **Skipping Meals**

    - Missing meals might make you extremely hungry later, leading to overeating. Balanced meals keep you on track.

3. **Eliminating Entire Food Groups**

    - Cutting out all carbs, fats, or proteins can cause imbalances. Rather than removing a whole group, choose healthier versions within each group.

4. **Comparing with Others**

    - Everyone's body is different. What works for a friend might not work for you. Focus on personal progress.

---

## How Sleep and Stress Affect Weight

1. **Sleep**

    - Lack of sleep can change hormones that regulate hunger, leading to cravings and overeating.

- Aim for 7-9 hours of quality sleep each night if possible.

2. **Stress Management**

    - Chronic stress triggers the release of cortisol, which can encourage the body to store fat, especially around the waist.

    - Activities like meditation, gentle exercise, or hobbies can help manage stress levels.

---

## Examples of Balanced Daily Eating for Weight Control

Here is a sample day for someone aiming to maintain or slightly reduce weight, depending on portion sizes:

- **Breakfast (7:00 AM)**

    - Whole-grain cereal with low-fat milk and fresh berries

    - A boiled egg or a small portion of cottage cheese

    - Water or unsweetened tea

- **Lunch (12:30 PM)**

    - Salad with grilled chicken (or beans), plenty of vegetables, and a light dressing

    - A piece of whole-grain bread on the side

    - Water

- **Afternoon Snack (3:30 PM)**
    - Apple with a tablespoon of peanut butter, or low-fat yogurt
    - Water

- **Dinner (6:30 PM)**
    - Brown rice with stir-fried vegetables (broccoli, peppers, onions) and shrimp or tofu
    - A drizzle of low-sodium soy sauce or your favorite herbs for flavor
    - Water

- **Optional Evening Snack (8:30 PM)**
    - A small handful of almonds or a few whole-grain crackers if hungry
    - Herbal tea or more water

Portion sizes should match your personal energy needs. Always tune in to hunger and fullness signals rather than forcing yourself to clean the plate.

## When to Seek Professional Guidance

1. **Major Weight Changes**

    - If you have gained or lost a significant amount of weight quickly and do not know why, a doctor can help identify possible health concerns.

2. **Long-Term Struggles**

    - If you have tried healthy approaches but see no progress or keep cycling up and down in weight, a registered dietitian or nutritionist can design a custom plan.

3. **Health Conditions**

    - Diabetes, thyroid disorders, or digestive issues can affect weight. Proper testing and advice can ensure you handle these conditions correctly.

---

## Staying Motivated for the Long Haul

Keeping weight under control is not a short project but a lifetime approach:

1. **Set Clear, Reasonable Goals**

    - Maybe you want to fit into a certain clothing size or have the endurance to run a local 5K. Having tangible targets helps keep you focused.

2. **Reward Yourself Without Food**

    - If you reach a milestone, treat yourself to something like a new workout outfit, a relaxing massage, or a fun outing instead of a huge dessert.

3. **Find a Support System**

    - Friends, family, or online groups can share tips, celebrate successes, and understand struggles.

    - Exercising with a partner can make it more enjoyable and keep you accountable.

4. **Look at the Bigger Picture**

    - A day of overeating or an unexpected setback does not undo all your progress. Focus on your overall patterns and keep moving forward.

## Conclusion of Chapter 14

Supporting weight control is about building daily habits that help you reach and maintain a healthy balance for your body. Rather than chasing quick fixes, you can rely on balanced meals, mindful portion sizes, steady physical activity, and a calm approach to stress and emotions. Whether you need to lose some weight, gain a bit, or just hold steady, small, consistent actions create lasting change. Stay in tune with your body's signals of hunger and fullness, pick nutrient-dense foods, and find ways to keep moving in your daily life. Over time, these steps add up to a more comfortable weight, improved confidence, and a stronger sense of well-being.

# CHAPTER 15

## Building a Strong Heart and Body

A healthy heart is like the engine of your body. It pumps blood that carries oxygen and nutrients to every cell. When your heart is strong, your entire body functions better, and you have more energy for the things you love. In this chapter, we will explore how to support a healthy heart and a strong body through a thoughtful way of eating, regular activity, and smart daily habits.

## Why Heart Health Matters

1. **Central Role in Blood Circulation**
   The heart sends oxygen-rich blood to your muscles, organs, and tissues. When the heart is in good shape, blood can flow easily, delivering nutrients and picking up waste.

2. **Long-Term Well-Being**
   Taking care of your heart can lower the chance of problems like high blood pressure or other heart concerns. A healthy heart often means a better chance of staying active, even as you get older.

3. **Better Daily Life**
   When your heart is strong, activities like climbing stairs, playing sports, or going for walks feel easier. You may notice you do not get out of breath so quickly.

4. **Supports Other Body Parts**
   The heart works together with your lungs, blood vessels, muscles, and even your brain. If your heart pumps well, these other parts of your body can do their jobs more efficiently.

# The Role of Food in Heart Health

What you eat plays an essential role in supporting your heart. Different types of foods affect your blood vessels, blood pressure, and the balance of fats in your bloodstream.

1. **Balancing Fats**

    - **Unsaturated Fats:** Foods like avocados, nuts, seeds, and oily fish (like salmon) contain fats that can be helpful for heart health. These fats may support normal cholesterol levels if you have them in moderate amounts.

    - **Saturated Fats:** Often found in butter, high-fat meats, and certain dairy products. Having too many foods with a lot of saturated fat can affect your heart if repeated all the time.

    - **Trans Fats:** These are in some processed or fried foods. These can be hard on your heart, so it is best to keep them low or avoid them completely.

2. **Watching Sodium**

    - Too much sodium (found in salt) can lead to higher blood pressure. High blood pressure can strain your heart over the years.

    - Try to choose fresh or minimally processed items, and check labels on packaged foods for sodium content. You can use flavor boosts like herbs, garlic, lemon juice, or vinegar instead of adding too much salt.

3. **Eating Enough Fruits and Vegetables**

    - Fruits and veggies have vitamins, minerals, and other natural compounds that may support a healthy heart.

    - They also offer fiber, which helps maintain normal blood cholesterol levels and digestion. Aim for a variety of colors, like red peppers, green spinach, and orange carrots, to get a wide range of nutrients.

4. **Choosing Heart-Friendly Proteins**

    - Lean meats (like chicken or turkey without the skin) can be part of a balanced plan. Fish, especially fatty fish like salmon or mackerel, provide omega-3 fats that can help your heart.

    - Plant proteins (beans, lentils, tofu, or tempeh) give you fiber and other nutrients without too much saturated fat.

    - Low-fat dairy or plant-based milk that has added calcium can help you get protein, but be mindful of added sugars in flavored varieties.

5. **Whole Grains**

    - Brown rice, oats, and whole wheat bread are examples of whole grains that have more nutrients and fiber than refined grains.

    - Fiber in whole grains helps balance cholesterol. It also leaves you feeling full so you may be less tempted to overeat.

# Keeping Blood Pressure in Check

Blood pressure is the force of blood pushing against your blood vessel walls. If it rises too high for too long, it can harm blood vessels and make your heart work harder than normal.

1. **Reducing Excess Salt**

    - Cooking most meals at home lets you control how much salt goes in. Restaurant meals and packaged snacks can be high in sodium.

    - Using spices and herbs instead of salt can give your food taste without risking too much sodium.

2. **Eating More Potassium**

    - Potassium helps balance the effects of sodium in your body. Good sources include bananas, potatoes, beans, tomatoes, and dark leafy greens.

    - Including these foods can support normal blood pressure.

3. **Staying Active**

    - Even moderate exercise, such as brisk walking, playing outside, or biking, can help your heart pump more effectively. Over time, this may keep blood pressure in a healthier range.

4. **Maintaining a Healthy Weight**
    - Carrying extra weight can place more load on your heart. On the other hand, being underweight is not helpful either. A balanced weight for your height can help your heart work better.

---

## Fiber's Role in Heart Health

Fiber helps your body manage cholesterol and supports a healthy digestive system:

1. **Soluble Fiber**
    - This type of fiber partially dissolves in water, forming a gel-like substance. It can "trap" some cholesterol in the digestive tract, helping remove it from your body.
    - Foods high in soluble fiber include oats, beans, lentils, apples, and citrus fruits.

2. **Insoluble Fiber**
    - This type helps food move through your digestive system. It keeps you "regular" and can prevent constipation.
    - Found in whole wheat bread, brown rice, and many vegetables.

3. **Combining Both Types**
    - Many plant foods contain both kinds of fiber. By eating a wide range of fruits, vegetables, whole grains, beans, and nuts, you get the benefits of both.

# Physical Activities for a Strong Heart

While nutrition is a major piece of the puzzle, exercise also matters:

1. **Aerobic Exercises**

   - Activities that raise your heart rate, such as running, brisk walking, biking, or swimming. These exercises train your heart to pump more effectively.
   - Even dancing can be aerobic if it makes your heart beat faster.

2. **Strength Training**

   - Lifting weights or doing bodyweight exercises (like push-ups or squats) can support your heart indirectly by building muscle. Stronger muscles use energy more effectively, which can help keep your weight in balance and reduce stress on your heart.

3. **Daily Movement**

   - You do not have to run a marathon. Simply walking more, taking the stairs, or doing chores around the house counts as daily movement. These smaller efforts can add up if you do them regularly.

4. **Rest and Recovery**

   - Your body, including your heart, needs time to recover from activity. Getting enough sleep and mixing active days with days of lighter movement helps avoid strain.

## Stress and Heart Health

Stress can affect your heart if it becomes overwhelming:

1. **How Stress Impacts the Body**

    - Stress hormones can affect blood pressure and your heart's workload. Over time, chronic stress might contribute to heart-related issues.

2. **Managing Stress**

    - Activities like gentle stretching, going for a calm walk, or practicing simple deep breathing can help you relax. Talking with friends or loved ones about your worries may also reduce tension.

3. **Avoiding Stressful Eating Habits**

    - Some people reach for sugary or salty snacks when anxious. This can lead to overindulgence in foods that do not help your heart. Instead, keep healthier snacks on hand or find a non-food way to feel better, such as reading a book or listening to music.

---

## The Role of Weight in Heart and Body Strength

1. **Not Too Heavy, Not Too Light**

    - Weighing too much puts extra strain on your heart and joints.

- Being very underweight can also cause problems, such as feeling tired and lacking enough nutrients for strong muscles.

2. **Finding Your Personal Balance**

    - Everyone has a different shape and size that is right for their health. Focusing on good nutrition and regular movement can guide you toward a weight that supports your heart.

3. **Eating Regular, Balanced Meals**

    - Skipping meals or extreme diets can stress your body. Instead, steady meals with protein, carbs, healthy fats, plus fruits and veggies, can help you stay energetic and strong.

---

## Making Heart-Healthy Choices at Any Age

1. **Children and Teens**

    - Encouraging an early pattern of eating more fruits and veggies, and making physical play a normal part of life, can build strong hearts from a young age.

    - Limiting sugary drinks and too many salty snacks is also helpful.

2. **Adults**

    - Adult schedules can be busy, but taking the time for balanced lunches, daily walks, or weekend hikes can protect your heart even with a hectic routine.

- Checking in with a doctor about blood pressure or cholesterol, especially if heart issues run in the family, can be wise.

3. **Older Adults**

    - Physical activities may need to be gentler, but continuing to move is important for heart strength.
    - Nutrient-dense foods become even more critical if appetites change with age.

## Smart Beverage Choices

What you drink can also influence your heart:

1. **Water**

    - The best choice for daily hydration. Keeping your blood volume balanced helps your heart pump effectively.
    - Aim to sip water throughout the day rather than waiting until you feel very thirsty.

2. **Herbal Teas**

    - Many are hydrating and can provide a calming break without extra calories or caffeine.
    - Avoid loading them with sugar or creamers that could add unhealthy fats or too much sweetness.

3. **Caffeine**

    - Moderate amounts of coffee or tea are usually fine for many people, but too much caffeine can speed your heart rate or disrupt sleep. Everyone's tolerance is different, so notice how your body reacts.

4. **Sugary Beverages**

    - Soda, fruit punch, and some sports drinks can have large amounts of sugar. Too much sugar can affect weight and heart health over time.

---

## Healthy Eating Patterns for a Strong Heart

Some people follow specific patterns to focus on heart health:

1. **Mediterranean-Style Plans**

    - Often emphasizes fruits, vegetables, whole grains, beans, nuts, seeds, and fish. Uses olive oil as the main fat. This pattern can benefit heart health when combined with an active lifestyle.

2. **DASH (Dietary Approaches to Stop Hypertension)**

    - A plan that is high in fruits, veggies, whole grains, and low-fat dairy. It limits foods high in saturated fat and sugar. Many find it helpful for keeping blood pressure in check.

3. **Plant-Focused Meals**

    - Not necessarily vegetarian, but meals that center around beans, lentils, whole grains, and vegetables, while cutting back on red meats. This can keep saturated fat levels lower and give you lots of fiber.

Remember, these are broad examples. You can blend ideas from different plans to fit your personal tastes and needs.

---

## Heart-Healthy Cooking Methods

1. **Grilling or Baking**

    - Helps reduce the amount of added fats in the cooking process, compared to deep-frying.

2. **Steaming or Boiling**

    - Great for vegetables, keeps their nutrients without adding fat. You can add flavors with herbs and spices afterward.

3. **Stir-Frying**

    - Uses only a small amount of oil if done right. Works well with lean protein, lots of vegetables, and whole-grain noodles or brown rice.

4. **Using Herbs and Spices**

    o   Rosemary, thyme, basil, garlic, onion, and many others can create interesting flavors. This can help you avoid relying too much on salt or sauces that are high in sugar.

---

## Common Myths About Heart Health

1. **Myth:** "You have to stop eating any fats for a healthy heart."
   **Truth:** Some fats (like unsaturated fats) are actually supportive for heart health. It is mainly trans fats and too many saturated fats that can pose problems if consumed too often.

2. **Myth:** "I am young, so I do not need to worry."
   **Truth:** Heart health starts early. Building good habits as a child, teen, or young adult can protect you later. It is easier to keep a strong heart than to fix problems that appear after many years.

3. **Myth:** "Only people who are very heavy develop heart troubles."
   **Truth:** Weight is one factor, but stress, genetics, salt intake, and a lack of exercise can also affect heart health. Even people with a moderate weight can face heart issues if they make unbalanced choices or rarely move.

4. **Myth:** "All cholesterol is bad."
   **Truth:** Your body needs some cholesterol to function. The concern arises when certain cholesterol levels in the blood become too high, combined with other factors like high blood pressure or excess weight.

# Practical Tips to Strengthen Your Heart

1. **Walk More Often**

    - If possible, walk to nearby places instead of driving. Use the stairs instead of the elevator when you can. Small decisions like these keep your heart active.

2. **Plan Balanced Meals**

    - Think of your plate: half fruits and veggies, a quarter for lean protein, and a quarter for whole grains. Add a small amount of healthy fats if needed (like a spoonful of olive oil or a sprinkle of seeds).

3. **Limit Processed Foods**

    - Many packaged snacks, frozen dinners, and fast foods come with extra salt, trans fats, or sugar. Having them once in a while might be okay, but not every day.

4. **Keep Portions Appropriate**

    - Even healthy meals can become too large. Be mindful of how hungry you truly are and eat slowly. Stopping when you feel content (not stuffed) can help with managing weight and supporting heart health.

5. **Routine Check-Ups**

    - Sometimes, a person might not notice small changes in blood pressure or cholesterol. Regular check-ups with a health professional can spot signs early.

## Linking a Strong Heart to a Strong Body

Having a strong heart is connected to the overall strength of your body in many ways:

1. **Efficient Oxygen Delivery**

   - If your heart pumps well, your muscles get the oxygen they need, boosting endurance in sports or daily tasks.

2. **Better Recovery**

   - After physical effort, a strong heart helps remove waste products from muscles more quickly. This can reduce soreness and support faster recovery.

3. **Improved Mental Clarity**

   - The brain benefits from good blood flow as well. Feeling mentally alert and focused often goes hand in hand with a healthy cardiovascular system.

4. **Stamina in Routine Activities**

   - Carrying groceries, gardening, or playing with kids might feel less tiring. A strong heart and body let you be active without feeling exhausted too soon.

---

## Children and Heart Health

Starting good habits at a young age sets the stage for lifelong wellness:

1. **Encourage Play**

    o   Children naturally enjoy running, jumping, or playing sports. This movement gives their hearts a gentle workout.

    o   Limit long periods of screen time when possible. Even short breaks for stretching or dancing can help.

2. **Balanced Family Meals**

    o   Involve kids in simple tasks like washing vegetables or measuring ingredients. Children who help prepare meals may be more willing to try new healthy foods.

3. **Positive Examples**

    o   If parents or older siblings make daily walks, bike rides, and balanced meals normal, children often learn to do the same.

---

## Checking In on Your Progress

When working on heart and body strength, it is helpful to see how you are doing:

- **Notice Changes in Breathing**: Do you become less short of breath when climbing stairs or doing chores?

- **Observe Energy Levels**: Are you feeling more energetic? Do you recover more quickly after playing sports or exercising?

- **Review Food Choices**: Are you including more fruits, vegetables, whole grains, and lean proteins? Are you reducing high-salt or high-sugar items?

- **Monitor Mood and Stress**: Sometimes, feeling calmer or sleeping better can be signs that your routine is helping your heart and body.

---

## Overcoming Challenges

1. **Busy Schedules**

   - If you have little time, try quick meals with simple ingredients like canned beans, frozen veggies, or a piece of fruit plus yogurt. Ten or fifteen minutes of brisk walking still counts as exercise.

2. **Budget Limits**

   - Budget-friendly items like beans, lentils, oats, eggs, and seasonal produce can keep your heart strong without spending too much. These foods are often more affordable than processed snacks.

3. **Lack of Motivation**

   - Team up with a friend for walks or cooking healthy meals together. Having someone else along can make you more likely to stick to a plan.

   - Set small goals, like trying one new veggie recipe each week or adding an extra 2,000 steps a day.

4. **Tempting Treats**

    - It is okay to enjoy sweets or salty snacks sometimes. Balance them with overall healthy meals and portion control.

    - If you have trouble with certain foods, consider not buying large amounts or keep them for special days.

---

## Celebrating Small Victories

Improving your heart health is a long-term process, so it is important to be proud of small steps:

- **Managed to Eat an Extra Serving of Veggies?** Great!

- **Swapped Sugary Drinks for Water a Few Times This Week?** That is progress!

- **Took a 15-Minute Walk After Dinner Each Day?** Your heart appreciates it.

Each positive choice adds up over weeks and months, shaping a stronger heart and body that can carry you forward.

---

# CHAPTER 16

## Keeping Energy Levels Steady

---

Feeling energetic helps you stay alert in school or at work, enjoy exercise, play with friends or family, and focus on your hobbies. Many people struggle with sudden energy drops or "crashes" during the day. Luckily, food choices, daily habits, and a bit of planning can help your body maintain steadier energy levels. In this chapter, we will look at ways to avoid big highs and lows in energy so you can stay balanced from morning until night.

---

## Understanding Energy in the Body

1. **What Is Energy?**

    - Your body's energy comes from calories in the foods and drinks you have. These calories get changed into fuel that helps you move, think, and keep body systems running.

2. **Types of Fuel**

    - Carbohydrates are usually the first source of quick energy, especially for your brain.

    - Proteins and fats give more lasting energy, though fats are used more slowly.

    - Vitamins and minerals do not directly provide energy (no calories), but they help your body use the energy from carbs, fats, and proteins effectively.

3. **Energy Balance**

    - If you consume many more calories than you burn, you might store excess energy as fat.

    - If you burn more than you eat, you may feel tired and start to lose weight. For steady energy, aim for a balance that fits your activity level.

---

## The Problem with Energy Highs and Lows

1. **Sugar Crashes**

    - Eating a lot of sugar can cause a sudden burst of energy. After that burst, blood sugar levels can quickly drop, leaving you feeling drained or restless.

    - Snacks like candy bars, sugary cereals, or sweet drinks can lead to a short spike and then a slump.

2. **Skipping Meals**

    - Missing breakfast or lunch may save time, but it can leave you feeling tired and more likely to overeat at the next meal. Large swings in hunger can cause swings in energy, too.

3. **Too Much Caffeine**

    - Drinks like coffee, tea, or energy beverages can give a fast jolt. But when caffeine wears off, you might feel more tired. Some people also get jittery or have trouble sleeping if they have too much caffeine or consume it too late in the day.

# Building a Daily Eating Pattern for Steady Energy

1. **Start with Breakfast**

   - After a night's sleep, your blood sugar is usually low. A balanced breakfast can restock your energy and help you stay focused.

   - Include complex carbohydrates (oats, whole wheat toast), protein (eggs, yogurt, nut butter), and maybe a piece of fruit or some vegetables. This mix steadies energy rather than causing spikes.

2. **Time Your Meals and Snacks**

   - Eating every few hours can help keep blood sugar from dropping too low, which can leave you feeling shaky or faint.

   - Plan small, nutritious snacks like a piece of fruit with nuts, or whole-grain crackers with low-fat cheese. This avoids sudden hunger that might lead to poor food choices later.

3. **Balance Protein, Carbs, and Fats**

   - A meal with only carbohydrates (like a bowl of plain pasta) might cause your energy to spike then crash. If you add lean protein and a bit of healthy fat, you get more stable energy.

   - Example: Whole-grain pasta with chicken and a bit of olive oil sauce plus veggies.

4. **Include Fiber**

    - High-fiber foods like vegetables, fruits, beans, and whole grains slow how fast your body absorbs sugar. This helps avoid sharp highs and lows in your energy.

---

## Smart Choices for Stable Energy

1. **Complex vs. Refined Carbohydrates**

    - **Complex Carbohydrates:** Found in whole grains, beans, and many vegetables. They break down more slowly, providing gradual energy.

    - **Refined Carbohydrates:** White bread, pastries, sugary cereals, and white rice are absorbed faster. They can lead to quicker energy spikes. Choose them less often or combine them with protein or fats to slow absorption.

2. **Protein's Role**

    - Protein helps fix tissues and stabilize energy levels because it digests more slowly than simple carbs. Having some protein at each meal (like fish, eggs, beans, or lean meat) can keep you feeling awake and focused.

3. **Healthy Fats in Moderation**

    - Avocados, nuts, seeds, and fatty fish (salmon) have fats that are better for your body. Fats take longer to digest, which can help steady energy.

        - However, do not go overboard. Too much fat at once might make you feel sluggish.

4. **Mindful Snacking**

    - If you need a snack, pick something with a combination of protein and carbs, such as apple slices with nut butter, or yogurt with berries. This helps keep energy stable between meals.

---

## Role of Hydration in Energy

1. **Water for Alertness**

    - Dehydration can make you feel tired or dizzy. Even mild dehydration sometimes feels like fatigue or difficulty focusing.

    - Sip water regularly, and pay attention to signs like dark-colored urine or dry lips, which suggest you might need more fluids.

2. **Electrolytes**

    - If you sweat a lot during exercise, you lose electrolytes like sodium, potassium, and magnesium. Replacing them through balanced meals (or a sports drink if the workout is intense) can help keep you energized.

    - Coconut water or low-sugar sports drinks can be options, but often water and a meal with enough minerals are enough for everyday activity.

3. **Caffeine and Other Drinks**

    - Moderation is key. A small cup of coffee or tea can give a boost. Too much might lead to a crash later or interfere with sleep, which then affects next-day energy.

    - Avoid turning to sugary drinks for a quick pick-me-up. They can cause the same crash problem as eating sugary foods.

---

## Physical Activity and Energy Levels

Exercise affects energy in positive ways:

1. **Better Blood Flow**

    - When you move, blood carries oxygen more efficiently. Over time, this can increase your overall energy and stamina.

2. **Mood and Alertness**

    - Physical activity can raise levels of certain chemicals in your body that help you feel good and awake. Even a short walk might help if you are feeling sluggish.

3. **Improved Sleep**

    - Regular exercise can lead to better rest at night. Good sleep is crucial for steady energy during the day.

4. **Caution with Overtraining**

    - Going too hard without enough rest can cause tiredness rather than boosting energy. Balance exercise days with lighter activity or rest days for recovery.

---

## Sleep's Critical Role

1. **Quality Sleep**

    - Your body fixes and refuels itself while you sleep. Not sleeping enough can make you feel tired, cranky, and less focused.

    - Aim for 7-9 hours if you are an adult, and even more if you are a teen or younger.

2. **Timing**

    - Going to bed and waking up at roughly the same times helps regulate your internal clock.

    - A bedtime routine—like reading or dimming lights—can guide your body to wind down naturally.

3. **Avoid Big Meals or Caffeine Late at Night**

    - Eating a huge dinner right before bed can disrupt sleep. If you are hungry at night, a small, light snack is better than a heavy meal.

- Caffeine too close to bedtime can keep you awake, leading to lower-quality rest and lower energy the next day.

## Handling Stress and Emotions for Consistent Energy

1. **Stress and Energy**

    - Worries and tension can drain you. Your body stays on alert, which can disrupt sleep and leave you feeling exhausted.

2. **Finding Healthy Outlets**

    - A short walk, a relaxed conversation with a friend, or writing in a journal can help let go of stress.

    - Taking breaks during work or study sessions helps refresh your mind.

3. **Avoiding Emotional Eating**

    - Some people turn to high-sugar, high-fat foods when stressed. This might lead to a fast energy boost but then a drop. Try non-food ways to feel better, such as breathing exercises or listening to calming music.

# Planning Ahead for Steadier Days

1. **Meal Prep**

    - Cooking a batch of whole grains, grilling lean protein, and washing vegetables in advance lets you build balanced meals easily.

    - This way, you avoid the temptation to grab quick but less healthy options when you are hungry.

2. **Packing Snacks**

    - Keep portable, balanced options like small bags of nuts, whole-grain crackers, or dried fruit handy.

    - This can stop you from having to buy candy or chips when hunger strikes away from home.

3. **Setting Routine**

    - Try to eat breakfast, lunch, and dinner around the same times daily. Add one or two small snacks if needed.

    - Predictable meal times help your body know when to expect fuel.

# Different Age Groups and Energy

1. **Children**

    - Kids have high energy needs for growth and play. Skipping meals can lead to crankiness or trouble focusing at school.

    - Balanced, kid-friendly snacks (like yogurt, fruit, veggie sticks) support their natural need for frequent fuel.

2. **Teens**
    - Teenagers often have growth spurts and busy schedules with sports or activities. They need more calories than some adults, but those calories should still come from wholesome foods rather than mainly from junk food or energy drinks.

3. **Adults**

    - Work or family responsibilities can lead to missed meals or reliance on quick fixes like coffee and sugary snacks. Maintaining a pattern of balanced meals helps avoid energy dips in the middle of the day.

4. **Older Adults**

    - Sometimes appetite decreases with age, but consistent nutrients are still important for stable energy. Softer foods or smaller meals spread through the day can help.

    - Staying hydrated is crucial, as thirst signals may weaken.

## How to Spot Hidden Energy Zappers

1. **Sugary Desserts**

    - Cakes, cookies, donuts. These taste good but can cause a fast spike in blood sugar, then a slump. If you want dessert, aim for a small portion or a fruit-based dessert.

2. **Stimulants Too Late**

    - If you have tea, coffee, or chocolate in the evening, it might mess up your sleep. That leaves you feeling drained tomorrow.

3. **Excess Screen Time**

    - Using phones, tablets, or computers near bedtime can keep your brain alert. The blue light from screens can trick your body into thinking it is daytime.

4. **Large Gaps Between Meals**

    - If you eat breakfast at 7 AM but do not have lunch until 2 PM, you might feel very hungry and tired mid-morning. A small snack at 10 or 11 can solve this.

---

## Tips for a Day with Balanced Energy

Below is an example of how to arrange meals and activities to keep energy more constant. Adjust times as needed:

- **Wake Up (6:30 AM)**
  - Drink a glass of water to hydrate.

- **Breakfast (7:00 AM)**
  - Whole-grain toast with peanut butter, a banana, and low-fat milk.
  - This combo has fiber, protein, and carbs to start the day.

- **Mid-Morning (10:00 AM)**
  - If hungry, have a small snack: yogurt with berries or a handful of almonds.
  - Drink water.

- **Lunch (12:30 PM)**
  - Brown rice bowl with grilled chicken, mixed veggies, and a light sauce.
  - Water to drink.

- **Afternoon (3:00 PM)**
  - Take a short walk or stretch if you feel sluggish.
  - Possible snack: whole-grain crackers with low-fat cheese.

- **Dinner (6:30 PM)**
    - Salmon (or bean stew if you prefer plant-based), whole-grain pasta or quinoa, plus roasted vegetables.
    - Water, or unsweetened tea, to stay hydrated.
- **Evening (8:00 PM)**
    - If you need a little more, have a small piece of fruit or some air-popped popcorn.
    - Avoid high-sugar or heavy snacks right before bed.
- **Wind Down (9:00 PM)**
    - Turn off bright screens, try reading or a quiet activity. Aim to get enough rest so you wake up refreshed.

---

## Avoiding the Afternoon Slump

Many people feel a drop in energy around 2 to 4 PM:

1. **Plan a Nutritious Lunch**
    - A meal that combines whole grains, lean protein, and vegetables is less likely to cause you to crash later.
2. **Short Movement Break**
    - Taking a short walk or stretching your legs can boost circulation and wake you up.

3. **Hydrate**

    - Sometimes, feeling tired can mean you need water. Keep a water bottle nearby.

4. **Healthy Snack**

    - If you are truly hungry, pick something like a small portion of nuts, low-sugar yogurt, or fresh fruit. Avoid big desserts that cause a sugar crash.

---

## Handling Shifts in Schedule

Busy days, travel, or special events can interrupt normal eating times:

1. **Be Flexible**

    - If you cannot eat a usual meal, look for a balanced option from a nearby café or carry a meal replacement bar that is not overloaded with sugar.

    - Keep healthy snack items in your bag or car to avoid a total energy meltdown.

2. **Travel Tricks**

    - If you are on a plane or train, pack nuts, dried fruits, or whole-grain sandwiches. Airport meals may be limited and high in salt or sugar.

3. **Listen to Your Body**

    - If you miss a meal, you may feel tired. Try to catch up with a balanced option soon, but do not overeat just because you are behind schedule.

---

## Special Considerations

1. **Physical Jobs or Intense Exercise**

    - People who do heavy labor or intense sports might need more calories, more protein, and more frequent snacks to keep energy steady.

    - Focus on nutrient-dense choices instead of sugary bars or candies.

2. **Medical Conditions**

    - Some conditions (like diabetes, thyroid imbalances, or chronic fatigue) can heavily affect energy. Following medical guidance for eating and medication is vital.

3. **Allergies or Dietary Restrictions**

    - If you cut out certain foods, make sure you find alternative ways to get the nutrients you need for energy. For example, if you do not eat dairy, find other calcium and protein sources.

---

## Mental Energy and Focus

1. **Brain Fuel**

    o The brain relies on steady blood sugar. Complex carbs and balanced meals help you avoid feeling foggy.

2. **Taking Breaks**

    o Working for hours without rest can lower mental energy. A quick stretch, a breath of fresh air, or a couple of minutes to close your eyes can recharge your mind.

3. **Avoiding Extreme Diets**

    o Diets that remove entire food groups or severely cut calories can leave you drained. Your brain needs a range of nutrients to function well.

---

## Tracking What Works for You

Everyone's body is a little different. Pay attention to:

- **Which Foods Give You Lasting Energy?** Maybe oatmeal in the morning keeps you going until lunchtime, or perhaps eggs and whole-grain toast works best.

- **Does a Certain Snack Help More Than Others?** You might find that an apple with peanut butter keeps you steady, while sugary cookies lead to a crash.

Keeping a simple note of how you feel after meals can guide you in making better choices. Over time, you can develop a personal routine that fits your life and keeps your energy more stable.

## Conclusion of Chapter 16

Keeping energy levels steady throughout the day helps you focus, feel strong, and enjoy activities without constant highs or lows. By choosing balanced meals that combine complex carbohydrates, protein, and healthy fats, as well as staying hydrated and managing stress, you can avoid many of the common pitfalls that lead to energy crashes. Pair these eating habits with regular physical movement and enough sleep to give your body the best chance for consistent energy. Remember that small, steady steps—like having a balanced breakfast or planning a nutritious afternoon snack—can make a big difference in how lively and alert you feel each day.

# CHAPTER 17

## Eating to Feel Good Inside and Out

Feeling good inside and out means taking care of both your body and your mind. The foods you eat can affect your mood, how your skin and hair look, and how well you handle stress. While no single food can solve every problem, choosing a variety of wholesome foods can help you feel calmer, happier, and healthier overall. In this chapter, we will explore how different nutrients support your mood, ways to keep your digestive system happier, and tips for feeling more confident in your own skin.

## How Food Affects Your Mood

You might notice that after a balanced meal, you feel more stable and content, while eating too many sweets might leave you jittery or tired later. This happens because the nutrients in foods can influence brain chemicals and energy levels.

1. **Steady Blood Sugar, Steady Mood**

    - When your blood sugar drops too low, you might feel cranky or have trouble focusing. Eating balanced meals with whole grains, protein, and healthy fats helps your body break down sugar more slowly, so you avoid big swings in mood.

    - Sugary treats and drinks can cause a quick rise in blood sugar, followed by a crash. This can make you feel suddenly tired or sad.

2. **Nutrients That Help the Brain**

    - **Omega-3 Fats:** Found in foods like salmon, sardines, and walnuts, can support brain function. Some research suggests they might assist with maintaining a calmer mood.

    - **B Vitamins:** Help the brain use energy and make certain chemicals for stable emotions. Foods like leafy greens, beans, and whole grains have B vitamins.

    - **Vitamin D:** Often called the "sunshine vitamin." Your body makes it from sunlight, but it is also in some foods (like fatty fish or fortified milk). Low levels can affect mood and energy.

3. **Proteins and Amino Acids**

    - Protein in foods like beans, eggs, fish, tofu, or lean meats breaks down into amino acids. Certain amino acids may help produce feel-good chemicals in the brain.

    - Balancing protein with other nutrients at each meal helps you feel steady and less prone to mood changes.

4. **Emotional Eating**

    - Many people eat snacks or desserts when they are upset or bored, trying to feel better. While an occasional treat is fine, turning to food every time you feel down can lead to guilt or poor nutrition.

- If you find yourself eating mostly because you are upset rather than hungry, try a different activity, like taking a walk, listening to music, or talking with a friend.

---

## Feeling Better from the Inside: Gut Health

Your gut (the digestive tract) is sometimes called a "second brain." It has nerves that communicate with your main brain. A healthier gut can support better overall well-being.

1. **What Is Gut Health?**

    - It means having a good balance of helpful bacteria in your digestive system. These bacteria help break down food and can produce substances that may affect mood and immunity.

    - If your gut is upset, you might notice bloating, discomfort, or changes in bowel habits.

2. **Foods That Support Gut Health**

    - **Fiber-Rich Foods:** Vegetables, fruits, whole grains, beans, and lentils feed helpful gut bacteria.

    - **Fermented Foods:** Yogurt with live cultures, kefir, sauerkraut, kimchi, and kombucha can add helpful bacteria (probiotics) to your system. Check labels to see if they have live cultures.

- **Avoid Too Much Junk Food:** Foods heavy in sugar, unhealthy fats, or additives may disturb the balance of bacteria in your gut if eaten too often.

3. **Stay Hydrated**
    - Drinking enough water helps move food through the digestive tract. This can lower the chance of constipation and keep your gut lining healthy.
    - Thirst can sometimes feel like hunger, so if you are unsure, try a glass of water first and see if that helps.

4. **Taking Care with Antibiotics**
    - Antibiotics kill harmful bacteria when you are sick, but they can also affect helpful gut bacteria. If you are on antibiotics, consider including foods with probiotics (like yogurt) or talk to a health professional for guidance.
    - Always finish antibiotic courses as directed by a doctor, but remember to support your gut with fiber and possibly probiotic foods.

---

## How Skin and Hair Reflect What You Eat

Healthy skin and hair rely on vitamins, minerals, protein, and adequate hydration.

1. **Proteins for Skin, Hair, and Nails**
    - Skin, hair, and nails are made of proteins like collagen and keratin. Eating enough protein-rich foods—like fish, beans, lentils, eggs, or lean meats—helps build and fix these tissues.

2. **Antioxidants**

    - Vitamins A, C, and E act as antioxidants. They protect cells from damage due to everyday stress and environmental factors. Fruits, vegetables, and nuts can offer these nutrients.

    - For example, bell peppers, strawberries, and oranges have vitamin C, which also aids in making collagen for healthy skin.

3. **Healthy Fats for Moisture**

    - Fats from avocados, nuts, seeds, and fatty fish help keep your skin soft and hair shiny. They also help the body absorb vitamins that support skin health.

    - Not having enough essential fats can contribute to dry skin or brittle hair.

4. **Water Intake**

    - Staying hydrated supports a healthy glow. Dryness or flakiness can be linked to not getting enough water. Even mild dehydration can affect skin appearance.

---

## Confidence and Body Image

Eating well helps you feel good physically, but it can also influence how you view yourself.

1. **Listening to Your Body**

    - Try to be aware of signs of hunger and fullness. Eating until you are just satisfied can help you avoid feeling too stuffed or hungry.

    - This self-awareness can lead to a more positive connection with food. Instead of labeling foods as "bad" or feeling guilty after eating, aim for balance.

2. **Avoid Crash Diets**

    - Fast or extreme diets might promise a quick change in how you look but can lead to weakness, hair problems, or mood changes. They do not usually produce lasting confidence if your body feels deprived.

    - Balanced, steady changes in eating habits can help your body find a healthy weight and shape naturally.

3. **Focusing on Health, Not Just Looks**

    - Feeling strong and energetic often improves your self-image more than any number on the scale.

    - Celebrate what your body can do—like running, dancing, or gardening—rather than only focusing on how it appears.

4. **Comparisons to Others**

    - Everyone has a different body type and metabolism. Comparing yourself to friends, family, or celebrities might lead to disappointment.

- It can help to set personal goals, like feeling more energized or improving at a certain exercise, rather than chasing someone else's looks.

## Foods That Support Calmness

Certain foods and eating patterns can help you handle stress better. Though they are not cures, they might contribute to a calmer mindset:

1. **Complex Carbohydrates**

    - Whole grains, beans, and vegetables provide a steadier flow of energy, helping avoid jittery feelings that come from sudden sugar spikes. A stable energy supply can lower stress.

2. **Magnesium-Rich Foods**

    - Leafy greens (spinach), nuts (almonds), seeds, and beans have magnesium. Low magnesium might be linked to increased feelings of tension.

    - Having enough of this mineral can help your muscles and nerves relax.

3. **Herbal Teas**

    - Teas like chamomile or peppermint (without added caffeine) can soothe you if you feel stressed. Sipping something warm can also be a comforting ritual at the end of the day.

4. **Moderate Caffeine**

    - Small amounts of caffeine may help you feel alert, but too much can cause restlessness or worry. If you notice you are more anxious after coffee, consider switching to decaf or herbal options, especially in the afternoon or evening.

---

## Boosting Self-Esteem Through Food and Activity

Feeling good is not just about the foods you eat. Physical activities and self-care also play big roles.

1. **Exercise and Endorphins**

    - Moving your body, whether dancing, swimming, or playing soccer, can release endorphins. These are chemicals that help you feel happier.

    - Regular activity works with good nutrition to help you feel stronger and more confident.

2. **Celebrating Progress**

    - If you manage to include more fruits and vegetables in your meals, that is a success. If you tried a new exercise, that is another win. Recognize your progress instead of pointing out flaws.

3. **Social Connections**

    - Sharing a meal with friends or family can help you feel supported. Cooking or eating together often brings joy and strengthens bonds.

4. **Mental Breaks**

    - Taking time each day to rest or do something fun helps reduce mental strain. Stress can make it harder to stick to balanced meals. When you feel relaxed, it is easier to choose foods that help your body and mood.

---

## Simple Strategies to Keep Feeling Good

1. **Plan Balanced Meals**

    - You do not need fancy recipes. Aim for a protein source, a vegetable or fruit, and a whole grain in most meals. Add healthy fats in small amounts.

2. **Avoid Extreme Hunger**

    - If you go too long without eating, you might feel shaky or irritable. A small, healthy snack can keep you level until the next meal.

    - Examples: Apple slices with peanut butter, a yogurt cup, or a handful of nuts and seeds.

3. **Mindful Eating**

    - Try to chew slowly, notice the flavors, and stop when you are satisfied. Rushing meals can lead to overeating or missing your body's signals.

    - This also makes mealtime more pleasant and helps you appreciate food.

4. **Keep Healthy Snacks Available**

    - If you have sliced vegetables, fruit, yogurt, or whole-grain crackers at home, you are more likely to pick those when hunger hits.

    - Limit how many bags of chips or boxes of cookies you keep around. If you have treats, that is okay, but hide them so they are not the first thing you see.

---

## Handling Emotions That Affect Eating

1. **Stress-Eating**

    - Stress can cause cravings for sweet or salty foods. Instead of immediately reaching for chips or candy, pause and ask, "Am I hungry or just stressed?" If it is stress, try a quick walk or talk with a friend.

2. **Boredom-Eating**

    - Sometimes you eat just because you have nothing else to do. Fill those moments with a hobby, a puzzle, or a phone call to a friend.

    - Having a glass of water or a piece of fruit might be enough if you are only a bit hungry.

3. **Sadness-Eating**

    - When feeling down, you might want comforting treats. It can help in the short term, but too much can lead to guilt later. If you need comfort, consider journaling or listening to calming music before heading to the fridge.

4. **Celebrating with Food**

    o   We often celebrate birthdays or holidays with big meals or sweets. That is fine, but remember to include some healthy dishes, too. Balance a slice of cake with vegetables or fruit on the side.

---

## Building Positive Habits Step by Step

1. **Set Realistic Goals**

    o   Rather than trying to change everything at once, pick one or two habits to work on—like adding one extra vegetable serving daily or swapping soda for water most days.

    o   Each small success makes you feel more confident and leads to better overall habits.

2. **Check in with Yourself**

    o   After a week or two, ask yourself how you feel. More energetic? Calmer? Are you sleeping better? Recognizing these benefits can motivate you to keep going.

3. **Be Kind to Yourself**

    o   Some days you may eat more junk food or skip exercise. It happens. Learn from it rather than beating yourself up. Think about what you can do differently next time.

4. **Celebrate Non-Food Rewards**

    - If you accomplish a health goal, treat yourself to something that supports your well-being, like a new book, a scented candle, or a comfortable pair of shoes for walking.

---

## Sleep, Stress, and Feeling Good

1. **Quality Sleep**

    - If you sleep well, you often feel calmer and make better food choices the next day. Too little sleep can raise stress hormones, making you crave sugary snacks.

    - Aim for a consistent bedtime and a relaxing routine before you turn out the lights.

2. **Relaxation Techniques**

    - Short breathing exercises, gentle stretches, or writing down what you are thankful for can lower stress. Less stress can mean fewer urges to eat sweets for comfort.

3. **Avoid Technology Before Bed**

    - The bright light from phones or tablets can confuse your brain into thinking it is daytime. Try to switch off screens at least 30 minutes before sleep.

# Finding Joy in Healthy Eating

1. **Try New Recipes**

    - Sometimes, eating the same foods gets boring. Looking up simple recipes for vegetables, beans, or whole grains can spark excitement.

    - You might discover you love roasted cauliflower or lentil soup if you give them a chance.

2. **Use Herbs and Spices**

    - Flavors like basil, cilantro, garlic, ginger, or cinnamon can make simple dishes taste amazing without adding too much salt or sugar.

3. **Cook with Friends or Family**

    - Preparing meals together can be a fun social time. Younger family members can help wash produce or stir ingredients, learning healthy habits along the way.

4. **Present Food Nicely**

    - Arranging cut fruit in a colorful way or setting out vegetables in a bright pattern can make healthy meals more appealing. We often eat first with our eyes.

## Checking In on Changes

If you start adjusting your meals and snacks for better mood and well-being, keep track of how you feel:

1. **Mood Diary**

    - Write down what you eat and how you feel afterward. Do you feel more stable on days you have balanced meals? Do too many sweets make you crash? This can guide future decisions.

2. **Energy Levels**

    - Check if you still get mid-afternoon crashes or if you have more continuous energy from breakfast to bedtime. If you notice improvements, see what part of your diet changed.

3. **Sleep Quality**

    - If you begin eating more fiber and having fewer heavy meals close to bedtime, your sleep might get better. A restful night can boost how you feel the next day.

4. **Skin and Hair**

    - Changes might take time, but after a few weeks of eating more nutrient-rich foods, you could see improvements in skin clarity or hair texture. Keep in mind there are many factors, including genetics and weather, but nutrition can be a strong helper.

## Self-Care Beyond Food

Although eating well plays a big part in feeling good inside and out, you can combine it with other forms of self-care:

1. **Regular Activity**

    - Dancing, walking, or playing a sport can lift your mood, help circulation, and improve muscle tone.

2. **Creative Outlets**

    - Drawing, playing an instrument, or crafting can calm your mind and reduce stress eating.

3. **Social Support**

    - Spending time with friends and family (in person or through calls) can boost happiness and lower stress.

4. **Mind-Body Practices**

    - Activities like yoga, gentle stretching, or meditation can connect your breathing and body awareness, further supporting emotional balance.

# CHAPTER 18

## Managing Food Choices in Daily Life

Life can be busy and filled with distractions. From juggling work or school schedules to running errands and spending time with loved ones, it is easy to feel that healthy eating gets pushed aside. However, there are many simple strategies to help you manage your food choices, even on the busiest days. In this chapter, we will look at practical ways to handle grocery shopping, meal planning, eating out, special diets, and social situations, so you can maintain a balanced approach to nutrition.

## How to Plan and Shop Wisely

Planning can keep you from feeling stuck when hunger strikes. Good meal planning and smart shopping protect both your wallet and your health.

1. **Make a Meal Schedule**

    - Sketch out what you will eat for the week. It does not have to be detailed for every meal, but list a few main dishes.

    - Note the days when you have less time to cook. Plan something quick for those days, like a one-pot meal or a simple stir-fry.

2. **Create a Shopping List**

    - Write down the ingredients needed for your planned meals.

- Check your fridge and cupboards first, so you do not buy duplicates or miss important items.
- Stick to your list in the store to reduce impulse buys.

3. **Shop the Perimeter**

    - Fresh fruits, vegetables, meats, fish, dairy, and eggs are often found around the edges of the store.
    - Middle aisles hold packaged foods, which you might still need (like whole-grain pasta, beans, or canned tomatoes), but stay mindful of highly processed snacks.

4. **Choose More Whole Foods**

    - Whole fruits and vegetables, grains like brown rice or oats, and lean proteins are usually better than overly processed items.
    - Look for words like "whole grain," "low-sodium," or "no-sugar-added" on labels if you buy packaged items.

---

## Meal Prep for Busy Days

Even if you do not have a lot of time each day, a little prep can make meals easier.

1. **Batch Cooking**

    - Pick a day (like Sunday) to cook a large batch of grains (rice or quinoa), roast a tray of vegetables, or prepare protein (chicken, beans, or tofu).

- Store them in containers. Throughout the week, you can quickly assemble balanced meals with these ready-to-use items.

2. **Cut and Store Produce**

    - Wash and chop vegetables in advance. Keep them in clear containers in the fridge, so they are easy to see and use for salads, stir-fries, or quick snacks.

    - You are more likely to eat vegetables if they are already prepared.

3. **Cook Once, Eat Twice**

    - Make extra servings of dinner and use leftovers for lunch. For example, if you cook grilled chicken and steamed vegetables for dinner, save a portion to put over salad or rice for lunch.

4. **Use Your Freezer**

    - Freeze soups, stews, or cooked beans in individual portions. If you have a busy day, thaw and reheat one portion for a fast, nutritious meal.

    - Frozen fruits and veggies are also handy for quick smoothies or side dishes.

# Eating Well at Work or School

Long hours away from home can lead to hasty food choices, but planning can help.

1. **Pack Lunches and Snacks**

    - A simple lunch might be a sandwich on whole-grain bread with lean protein and vegetables, plus a piece of fruit.

    - Healthy snacks like nuts, yogurt, or cut-up veggies can keep hunger under control between meals.

2. **Keep Water Nearby**

    - Thirst can sometimes be mistaken for hunger. Having a water bottle at your desk or in your backpack encourages regular sips, helping you stay hydrated.

3. **Watch Out for the Vending Machine**

    - If you often rely on vending machines, try bringing your own snacks to avoid chips or candy bars.

    - If you do choose from a vending machine, look for nuts, seeds, or lower-sugar granola bars if available.

4. **Plan Breaks**

    - If your schedule allows, take a short walk at lunch or eat outside if the weather is good. A bit of sunshine and movement can refresh your mind and keep your body active.

# Making Good Choices at Restaurants

Dining out is fun and social, but restaurant meals can have lots of hidden calories, salt, or sugars. You do not have to avoid them; just be a bit mindful.

1. **Scan the Menu**

    - Look for words like "grilled," "baked," or "steamed." These cooking methods often use less added fat than "fried" or "smothered."

    - Soups that are broth-based instead of cream-based can be lighter.

    - If possible, check the menu online before you arrive, so you are not overwhelmed by too many choices.

2. **Portion Awareness**

    - Restaurant portions can be large. You can share a dish with a friend or ask for a take-home container right away, saving half for another meal.

    - If you start with a simple salad or broth-based soup, you may feel satisfied sooner.

3. **Smart Side Dishes**

    - Choose steamed vegetables, a side salad, or brown rice instead of fries. This adds fiber and nutrients without too much extra salt or fat.

- If you really want fries, consider splitting them with someone so you do not have a giant portion to yourself.

4. **Go Easy on Sugary Drinks**

    - Sodas, sweet tea, and flavored lemonades often have lots of sugar. Water, sparkling water, or unsweetened iced tea can be better everyday choices.

    - Save sweet drinks for special occasions if you like them, but keep the portion reasonable.

---

# Adapting to Special Diets

Some people follow certain eating patterns due to health needs, personal beliefs, or allergies. Here are a few common ones and how to handle them:

1. **Vegetarian or Vegan**

    - Focus on protein from beans, lentils, tofu, tempeh, nuts, seeds, and some whole grains.

    - Include a range of vegetables and fruits to get essential vitamins and minerals.

    - Check labels for hidden animal products if you are strict vegan.

2. **Gluten-Free**

    - If you cannot eat wheat, barley, or rye, choose alternatives like rice, corn, quinoa, or gluten-free oats.

    - Many packaged gluten-free foods can still be high in sugar or salt, so check labels carefully.

    - Whole foods like fruits, veggies, beans, meats, and fish are naturally gluten-free.

3. **Dairy-Free**

    - Look for calcium-fortified plant-based milks (almond, soy, oat) if you do not consume cow's milk.

    - Keep an eye on vitamin D and B12 levels if dairy is a main source for you. Fortified products can help fill this gap.

    - Yogurt made from coconut, soy, or almonds can be an option, but check for added sugars.

4. **Low-Sodium**

    - If you need to keep salt low, focus on fresh foods instead of packaged or canned items.

    - Use herbs, spices, vinegar, lemon, or garlic to add flavor without salt.

    - Rinse canned beans or vegetables under water to remove some sodium.

# Handling Social Events and Gatherings

Parties, holiday feasts, and celebrations often feature lots of sweet treats, fatty snacks, and sugar-filled drinks. You can still enjoy these events without giving up on healthier habits.

1. **Eat Before You Go**

    - Have a small balanced snack, such as fruit with yogurt or whole-grain toast with peanut butter, so you are not starving upon arrival.

    - This helps you avoid grabbing too many cookies or chips right away.

2. **Look for Healthier Options**

    - Many gatherings include fruit salads, veggie trays, or lean protein options. Fill part of your plate with these before sampling richer dishes.

    - You do not have to skip your favorite foods. Just balance them with lighter sides or smaller portions.

3. **Watch Sugary Drinks and Alcohol**

    - At celebrations, it is easy to drink more soda or juice than you realize. Try mixing sparkling water with a splash of juice for flavor.

    - Alcoholic drinks can have many empty calories and can lead to mindless snacking if you are not careful. If you choose to drink, do so in moderation, and sip water in between.

4. **Offer to Bring a Dish**

    - If the party is a potluck, contribute a healthy but tasty dish, like a colorful salad or vegetable-based appetizer. That way, you know there is at least one dish you can enjoy without worry.

---

## Eating on the Go and Traveling

When traveling for work or pleasure, fast food and convenience stores might feel like your only options, but you can plan ahead.

1. **Pack Snacks for the Journey**

    - Items like trail mix (nuts, seeds, a bit of dried fruit), whole-grain crackers, or fruit can keep you from buying candy or chips at gas stations or airport shops.

    - If driving, pack a small cooler with yogurt cups, baby carrots, or string cheese.

2. **Look for Balanced Options**

    - Many rest stops or airports have fruit cups, salads, or grilled sandwiches.

    - If you must choose fast food, go for grilled chicken or a small burger without extra sauces, and pick a side salad or fruit if possible.

3. **Stay Hydrated**

    - Long travel hours can dehydrate you. Keep a refillable water bottle and top it up whenever you can.

    - Avoid relying on soda or energy drinks, which might give a temporary lift but lead to a slump later.

4. **Plan for Language or Local Customs**

    - If visiting a new country, learning basic phrases to ask about ingredients or allergies can help you find suitable meals.

    - Exploring local produce markets can be a fun way to discover fresh fruits and vegetables.

---

# Technology and Eating Habits

Phones and computers are part of most people's daily routines. They can support or sabotage healthy eating depending on how you use them.

1. **Food Tracking Apps**

    - Some people find it helpful to log meals or track calories. This can show patterns, like too many evening snacks or not enough protein for breakfast.

    - Others might feel stressed by constant tracking. Decide if it motivates you or makes you anxious, and act accordingly.

2. **Recipe Apps and Websites**

   - You can find simple, healthy recipes online based on ingredients you have on hand. This can spark creativity and help you avoid takeout.

3. **Online Grocery Shopping**

   - Many stores let you order groceries online. This can reduce impulse buys if you stick to your virtual list. It can also save time if you are busy.

4. **Screen Time During Meals**

   - Watching videos or scrolling social media while eating might make you lose track of how much you have eaten. Try to focus on your meal for a few minutes.

   - This mindful approach can help you enjoy your food more and notice when you are full.

---

## Time-Saving Tips for Cooking

Not everyone loves to cook or has lots of time to do it. These ideas can help:

1. **One-Pan or One-Pot Meals**

   - Stir-fries, soups, or casseroles can include protein, vegetables, and grains all in one dish. You save time on both cooking and washing dishes.

2. **Microwave and Slow Cooker**

    - A slow cooker (or similar device) can cook meals while you handle other tasks. Toss in ingredients like beans, vegetables, and spices in the morning, and have dinner ready by evening.

    - Microwave steam bags for vegetables can be a quick way to cook them without losing many nutrients.

3. **Frozen Vegetables**

    - These are already washed and chopped, saving time. They are often flash-frozen at peak freshness, so they retain many vitamins.

    - Add them to soups, pasta sauces, or stir-fries.

4. **Simplify**

    - You do not have to make a fancy recipe every night. A meal of scrambled eggs, whole-grain toast, and sliced tomatoes can be done in minutes and still offer protein, fiber, and vitamins.

---

## Staying Motivated and Flexible

Sticking to balanced eating is easier when you allow for flexibility and accept that perfection is not the goal.

1. **Aim for Balance Most of the Time**

    - If you eat well most days, enjoying a slice of pizza or a dessert on occasion is unlikely to ruin your overall plan. Balance is about patterns over time, not single meals.

2. **Set Small, Realistic Goals**

    - Want to eat more vegetables? Start by adding one extra vegetable serving at dinner.

    - Want to reduce sugary drinks? Replace one daily soda with water and see how you feel, then continue from there.

3. **Adjust as You Learn**

    - Maybe you discover you have more energy when you eat protein in the morning. Or maybe you realize you are not a fan of certain veggies and need to find alternatives.

    - Keep experimenting to see what best fits your preferences, budget, and schedule.

4. **Plan for Breakdowns**

    - If you skip meal prep one week or have an especially busy day, do not beat yourself up. Just try to pick up healthy habits again as soon as you can.

    - Consistency over time matters more than one off day.

## Involving Family and Friends

Sharing healthy choices with the people around you can make it easier and more fun.

1. **Meal-Planning Together**

    - Ask family members or roommates what they would like to eat for the week. Rotate who chooses the main dish to keep it interesting.

    - Make a grocery list everyone can add to, then see if you can find healthier swaps for items that might be high in sugar or salt.

2. **Cooking as a Group**

    - Cooking with friends or family can turn meal prep into a social activity. You can teach each other new recipes or cooking tips.

    - Children can learn basic cooking skills, encouraging them to try fresh foods they helped prepare.

3. **Healthy Challenges**

    - You might do a 7-day challenge to add a fruit or vegetable to every meal, or cut down on sugary drinks for a week, sharing progress with friends.

    - Friendly competition can keep everyone motivated and engaged.

## Putting It All Together

Daily life gets busy, but you can develop strategies to keep up with balanced eating:

- **Plan Ahead:** Even a little meal planning can save time and stress.

- **Prep Foods in Batches:** Cook once, eat multiple times.

- **Be Mindful When Eating Out:** Choose grilled or baked dishes and watch portion sizes.

- **Adapt to Your Needs:** If you have a special diet, allergies, or limited time, look for foods and cooking methods that fit your life.

- **Stay Flexible:** Perfection is not required. Aim for steady habits that you can keep long-term.

---

## Conclusion of Chapter 18

Managing food choices in a busy world takes planning, creativity, and a willingness to adapt when things change. By making a simple meal schedule, shopping with a list, and preparing ingredients in advance, you can enjoy a range of balanced meals without feeling rushed. When dining out or at social events, small steps like choosing grilled over fried options or sharing a large dish can help you stay on track. Remember that long-term success comes from consistency, not from strict perfection. Every wise choice—like packing a healthy snack for school or picking a side of vegetables at a restaurant—helps you practice a balanced lifestyle. As you find a routine that works for your schedule, you will see how doable and satisfying it can be to manage your food choices in daily life.

# CHAPTER 19

## Nutritional Tips for All Ages

Different stages of life come with different needs. Children need meals that support growth, teenagers require enough energy to power busy schedules, adults balance work and health goals, and older adults focus on maintaining strength. In this chapter, we will look at suggestions for each age group, so you can adjust meals and snacks that fit the stage of life you or your loved ones are in. By keeping these guidelines in mind, you can help yourself and your family stay strong and feel well at every milestone.

## Infants and Toddlers (Ages 0-3)

**1. Breast Milk or Formula**

- For the first months, babies often rely on breast milk or formula. These contain essential nutrients for growth.

- If breastfeeding, pay attention to the mother's own diet. Her nutrient intake affects the quality of breast milk.

**2. Introducing Solid Foods**

- Around 6 months, many babies begin trying soft or pureed foods like mashed fruits, cooked vegetables, or baby cereals.

- Introduce single-ingredient foods one at a time, so you can watch for allergic reactions.

- Offer a variety of flavors and textures once they are ready. This can help them become more open to different foods later.

## 3. Important Nutrients

- **Iron:** Infants need enough iron for healthy brain development. Iron-fortified cereals or pureed meats can help as they begin eating solids.

- **Healthy Fats:** In early years, fats support brain growth. If they move on from formula or breast milk, full-fat dairy products can be helpful in moderation.

- **Hydration:** Babies get most fluids from milk (breast or formula) and, eventually, small sips of water when they start eating solid foods. Juice is not usually needed and can contribute excess sugar.

---

# Early Childhood (Ages 4-8)

## 1. Building Good Habits

- Kids learn by watching adults. If they see parents or siblings enjoy balanced meals, they often follow suit.

- Keep healthy snacks at eye level. If cut-up fruits or vegetables are in easy reach, they are more likely to pick them.

## 2. Balanced Plates

- Offer a variety of food groups: lean proteins (chicken, beans), whole grains (brown rice, whole wheat pasta), fruits, vegetables, and dairy (or dairy alternatives).

- Smaller stomachs might need smaller, more frequent meals. Offer three meals and one or two snacks per day if they get hungry between meals.

### 3. Limited Sugary Drinks

- Sodas, punches, and sweet teas can quickly add sugar without offering vitamins.

- Water or low-sugar milk alternatives are often better daily options.

### 4. Involving Them in Meal Prep

- Younger kids can wash fruits, add ingredients you have measured, or arrange veggie sticks on a plate.

- This early involvement can lead them to try more foods and enjoy the process of eating well.

---

## Tweens and Teens (Ages 9-18)

### 1. Growth Spurts

- Adolescents may grow quickly. They need enough protein, calcium, iron, and overall calories to support this.

- Encourage balanced meals, not just snacks or fast foods. While teens often prefer quick options, guiding them toward a mixture of protein, healthy fats, and complex carbs can help steady their energy.

### 2. Calcium for Bones

- Bones build mass in these years, which can affect lifelong bone strength.

- Dairy products (milk, yogurt), fortified dairy alternatives, leafy greens, and certain fish (like canned salmon with bones) can boost calcium intake.

### 3. Iron for Energy

- If iron is low, teens might feel tired or struggle to focus. Foods like lean meats, beans, lentils, spinach, and fortified cereals help.

- Pairing iron-rich foods with vitamin C (like oranges, tomatoes) can improve iron absorption.

### 4. Busy Schedules

- After-school activities, sports, and homework can lead to skipped meals or reliance on vending machines.

- Suggest portable snacks: whole-grain granola bars, trail mix (nuts, seeds, dried fruit), or cheese sticks. This way, they avoid going too long without proper fuel.

### 5. Handling Peer Pressure

- Teens might be swayed by trends like fad diets or skipping meals. Encourage a balanced view: no single food is all good or all bad. Moderation and variety matter.

- Remind them that fueling their body helps with sports, focus in class, and overall mood.

---

# Young Adults (Ages 19-30)

### 1. Independence in Eating

- Many young adults handle their own meals for the first time, like college students or those working full-time.

- Planning grocery lists and simple recipes helps avoid takeout or random snacks as main meals.

### 2. Balancing Work, Studies, and Health

- Busy lifestyles can lead to quick, processed foods or late-night dinners. Aiming for at least one balanced meal per day (with vegetables, lean protein, and a whole grain) is a good start.

- If cooking at home, using meal prep strategies (cooking once for multiple meals) can keep costs down and nutrition up.

### 3. Preventing Nutrient Gaps

- Calcium, iron, and vitamins might be overlooked if someone relies too much on packaged noodles, frozen pizza, or fast food.

- Adding a side salad or frozen vegetables to a quick meal can raise the nutrient level with minimal extra effort.

### 4. Physical Activity and Weight Management

- Some young adults notice changes in weight if they eat more junk food or become less active than they were as teenagers. Moderation is key.

- Routine exercise helps manage stress from work or school and keeps energy steadier.

# Midlife Adults (Ages 31-50)

**1. Maintaining Healthy Habits**

- With work, family, or community commitments, finding time to cook or exercise can be challenging.

- Setting realistic routines—like a 30-minute brisk walk at lunch and planning simple but balanced dinners—can help.

**2. Managing Stress Eating**

- Stress from jobs or caring for children (and sometimes aging parents) might tempt you to grab sweets or salty snacks.

- Try short breaks for breathing exercises, a quick chat with a friend, or a cup of herbal tea when tensions are high.

**3. Keeping Metabolism Active**

- Muscle mass can decline if not used. Eating enough protein and doing some strength-focused activity each week (like lifting weights or bodyweight exercises) helps preserve muscle.

- Consider including lean proteins (chicken, fish, beans) in most meals to repair and build muscle tissue.

**4. Eye on Heart Health**

- Blood pressure and cholesterol can start creeping up during these years. Lean meats, fish, whole grains, fruits, vegetables, and limiting excess sodium can support a healthy heart.

- Substituting sugary drinks with water or unsweetened tea also helps manage overall calorie intake.

# Older Adults (Ages 51 and Beyond)

### 1. Adjusting to Lower Calorie Needs

- Activity levels may dip with age, meaning fewer total calories might be required. Still, nutrient needs remain important or even increase.

- Focus on nutrient-dense foods: beans, lean proteins, fruits, vegetables, whole grains, and low-fat dairy (or fortified dairy substitutes).

### 2. Protein for Muscle Maintenance

- Muscle mass can decline over time, leading to frailty if not addressed. Including protein (eggs, fish, lean meats, beans) in meals helps keep muscles stronger.

- Splitting protein evenly across the day might benefit muscle repair.

### 3. Bone Health

- Bones weaken as people age, especially among women after menopause. Calcium and vitamin D become crucial.

- Getting enough dairy or fortified non-dairy options, plus safe sunlight exposure (for vitamin D), can help. In some cases, doctors may suggest supplements.

### 4. Staying Hydrated and Watching Fiber

- Thirst signals can be less noticeable with age. Drinking water regularly helps digestion and kidney function.

- Adding fiber from fruits, vegetables, whole grains, and beans helps avoid constipation and supports a healthy gut.

### 5. Possible Medication Interactions

- Some older adults take medications that affect how nutrients are absorbed. They might need guidance from a doctor or dietitian to avoid shortages or harmful interactions.

- For example, certain blood thinners can be affected by high vitamin K intake (found in leafy greens). Adjusting portion sizes under medical supervision can help.

---

## Special Considerations

### 1. Pregnancy and Breastfeeding

- Extra calories and nutrients, especially iron, folate, and calcium, are important during pregnancy.

- During breastfeeding, mothers need enough fluids and nutrient-rich meals to support milk production.

- Lean proteins, whole grains, fruits, vegetables, and healthy fats form a strong base. Check with a health professional for specific needs.

### 2. Chronic Illness

- Some conditions like diabetes, heart concerns, or celiac disease require careful attention to certain nutrients or food types.

- Working with a doctor or dietitian can create a meal plan that helps manage symptoms while still enjoying a variety of foods.

### 3. Food Allergies or Intolerances

- Children and adults alike can develop allergies (e.g., peanuts, tree nuts, eggs, wheat) or intolerances (e.g., lactose).

- Reading labels is key. Look for clear allergen warnings and consider safe substitutes like soy milk for cow's milk or seed butter for peanut butter.

---

## Tips for Making Family Mealtime Easier

### 1. One Meal for Everyone

- If each person wants a different meal, cooking becomes complicated. Finding crowd-pleasing dishes—like a baked chicken with vegetables on the side—lets individuals add their own toppings or seasoning.

- You can also serve meals "build-your-own" style: for example, taco night with various fillings and toppings.

### 2. Sharing Responsibilities

- Encourage older kids to help prep veggies or set the table. Younger ones can do small tasks like stirring (with supervision).

- Adults can rotate who cooks, who cleans up, or who shops. Splitting tasks makes it less stressful.

### 3. Balancing Preferences

- Maybe one child loves carrots, while another prefers peas. It is okay to offer two vegetable choices if it helps everyone enjoy dinner more.

- Over time, encourage tasting new items, but do not force large servings of disliked foods. Taste buds can change.

### 4. Creating a Positive Atmosphere

- Use mealtime to talk about the day, rather than focusing on the food battle. Avoid scolding about every bite.

- Fun conversations can make children more willing to try at least a few bites of new foods.

---

## Staying Active at Every Age

While this book focuses on nutrition, remember that activity complements good eating in staying healthy.

### 1. For Children

- Activities like riding a bike, dancing, or playing in a playground keep them moving and help direct their natural energy in a healthy way.

### 2. For Teens

- Joining sports teams or simply walking with friends can support heart and muscle health. Encourage them to explore what they enjoy—be it soccer, skateboarding, or casual jogging.

### 3. For Busy Adults

- Quick options like walking during a break, cycling to work, or following a short exercise video at home can fit into tight schedules.

- Making exercise a priority helps manage weight, reduces stress, and boosts mood.

### 4. For Older Adults

- Low-impact choices like gentle yoga, water aerobics, or short daily walks can keep joints and muscles in better shape.

- Strength exercises with light weights or resistance bands help maintain muscle mass.

---

## Overcoming Challenges at Different Life Stages

### 1. Children Who Are Picky Eaters

- Patience is key. Offer small portions of new foods alongside familiar items.

- Repeated exposure can help them accept new tastes. Avoid battles at the table; keep the mood calm and positive.

### 2. Teen Independence

- Teens might skip meals or buy junk food with friends. Suggest small steps, like carrying a healthy snack from home.

- Talk about how balanced meals can help with sports performance, energy, and clearer skin—benefits they might value.

### 3. Adults with Limited Time

- Use meal prep hacks: slow cookers, batch cooking, or combining fresh and frozen produce for quicker meals.

- If you can afford it, consider meal delivery kits that provide portioned ingredients. They may cost more but can save time and reduce stress.

### 4. Older Adults with Changing Appetites

- Smaller, more frequent meals might feel more comfortable if large meals seem overwhelming.

- Choose nutrient-dense foods so each bite counts, like oatmeal with nuts, soups loaded with beans and vegetables, or eggs with spinach.

---

## Budget-Friendly Tips for All Ages

### 1. Buy Seasonal Produce

- Fruits and vegetables in season usually cost less and taste better.

- Frozen or canned options (low-sodium, no-sugar-added) can be cheaper and last longer without spoilage.

### 2. Shop Sales and Bulk

- Beans, lentils, rice, and oats are often affordable sources of carbs, protein, and fiber.

- If you have space, buying family packs of meat or big bags of grains can lower the cost per serving.

### 3. Cook at Home

- Homemade meals often cost less than takeout. Plus, you control ingredients like salt and sugar.

- Simple recipes using basic ingredients can still taste great. You do not need fancy foods for balanced nutrition.

**4. Make Use of Leftovers**

- Turn leftover grilled chicken into a sandwich or salad the next day.

- Use leftover veggies in an omelet or soup. This cuts food waste and saves money.

## Small Changes That Have a Big Impact

No matter your age, little adjustments can make a big difference:

- **Add a Veggie to Each Meal:** Could be a handful of spinach stirred into soup or sliced cucumbers on the side.

- **Swap Sugary Drinks for Water:** Over time, you might lose the taste for very sweet beverages.

- **Try Whole-Grain Versions:** Whole-wheat bread, brown rice, or whole-grain pasta add fiber and nutrients.

- **Include Lean Protein at Breakfast:** An egg, a bit of leftover chicken, or peanut butter on toast can help stabilize energy.

- **Set Up Movement Breaks:** Even at older ages, a gentle stretch or walk helps circulation and mood.

# Handling Setbacks and Celebrations

### 1. Sick Days or Busy Days

- If you rely on quick packaged meals sometimes, do not stress. Get back to your routine when you can.

- Keep some pantry staples—like canned soup, canned tuna, or beans—on hand for emergency meals.

### 2. Special Events

- Birthdays, holidays, or family reunions often bring rich foods. Enjoy them in moderation and balance with lighter choices at other meals.

- If you go overboard one day, just return to your usual, balanced way of eating the next day.

### 3. Praise Efforts

- Whether you are praising a child for trying new fruits or congratulating yourself on making a healthier lunch, highlight positive steps.

- Encouragement keeps everyone motivated to continue or expand these habits.

## Staying Inspired Long-Term

1. **Variety Keeps Things Fresh**

    - Trying new recipes or cooking methods keeps meals from feeling boring.

    - Taste buds can shift over time, so foods you disliked before might become more appealing later.

2. **Set Achievable Goals**

    - Instead of saying "I will eat perfectly every day," aim to add an extra vegetable at dinner or reduce sugary snacks throughout the week.

    - Celebrate small wins to maintain momentum.

3. **Include Family and Friends**

    - Eating together can be fun and supportive. You can trade recipes, share meal prep duties, and encourage each other on days you feel less motivated.

4. **Focus on Feeling Good**

    - Pay attention to energy, mood, and how clothes fit more than numbers on a scale.

    - As you notice positive changes, that can strengthen your resolve to keep going.

# CHAPTER 20

## Putting It All Together

After exploring every facet of fitness and nutrition—from understanding basic nutrients to planning meals, choosing balanced snacks, supporting heart health, steadying energy, and learning tips for different life stages—we have covered a lot of ground. This final chapter will bring everything into a clear path forward. We will summarize the main ideas and give you a practical roadmap for continuing to build and sustain healthy eating patterns that support an active, fulfilling life.

## 1. Key Pillars of a Balanced Diet

Every chapter has highlighted certain principles that form a solid foundation:

### a. Variety

- Eating a wide range of foods—from colorful fruits and vegetables to whole grains, lean proteins, dairy or fortified alternatives, and healthy fats—helps you get the mix of nutrients your body needs.

- Different foods bring distinct vitamins, minerals, and flavors, keeping meals interesting and your diet well-rounded.

### b. Moderation

- Instead of labeling foods as "always good" or "always bad," look at how often you are having them and how much.

- You can still enjoy treats or richer meals if most of your choices center on nutrient-dense foods.

**c. Balance**

- In one meal, a balance of protein, carbohydrates, and a little fat prevents sharp spikes and drops in energy.

- Across the day, balancing heavier meals with lighter ones (or vice versa) keeps you on an even track.

**d. Hydration**

- Water is essential for nearly every process in your body. Staying hydrated helps digestion, energy levels, and even skin appearance.

- Aim to drink water throughout the day and rely less on sugary or heavily caffeinated beverages for hydration.

---

## 2. Understanding Nutrients in Simple Terms

Recall that macronutrients (proteins, carbs, and fats) supply energy, while micronutrients (vitamins and minerals) help your body work properly. Here is a quick review:

**a. Proteins**

- Build and fix muscles, organs, skin, and more.

- Aim to include a source of protein in each meal (e.g., beans, fish, eggs, lean meats, dairy, or dairy substitutes).

- Spreading out protein intake can help with muscle repair and steady energy.

### b. Carbohydrates

- Provide fuel for the body and brain.

- Choose complex carbs (whole grains, beans) more often than refined ones (white bread, pastries).

- Fruits and vegetables also offer carbs along with fiber, vitamins, and minerals.

### c. Fats

- Aid in absorbing certain vitamins, support hormone production, and offer stored energy.

- Unsaturated fats (olive oil, avocados, nuts) are generally more heart-friendly.

- Limit trans fats and keep an eye on saturated fats (high in butter, certain meats) for heart health.

### d. Vitamins and Minerals

- Support countless processes, from bone building (calcium, vitamin D) to immune function (zinc, vitamin C) to oxygen transport (iron).

- Eating a range of fruits, vegetables, whole grains, and proteins ensures you get a mix of these crucial nutrients.

---

## 3. Meal Planning Made Easier

### a. Start with Simple Meal Frameworks

- Begin each meal by thinking of a protein (beans, eggs, fish, poultry, lean meats, or dairy), add a whole grain (brown rice, whole wheat pasta, quinoa), and include at least one or two vegetables or a piece of fruit.

- This framework simplifies decisions and ensures you include the main food groups.

### b. Prepping or Cooking in Batches

- Choose a time during the week—maybe a weekend or a quieter evening—to make a large batch of grains, roast vegetables, or cook proteins. Refrigerate or freeze them in portions.

- This ready-to-use approach helps you quickly assemble meals on hectic days.

### c. Making Use of Leftovers

- If you are grilling chicken, consider cooking extra for salads or wraps the next day.

- Leftover vegetables can go into an omelet or a soup. Having pre-cooked ingredients means you can skip the takeaway line.

## 4. Snacking and Sweets in Check

### a. Smart Snacking

- It is fine to snack if you are genuinely hungry between meals. Pick snacks that have some protein or fiber, like yogurt with berries, nuts, or veggie sticks with hummus.

- Avoid snacking out of boredom or stress. A quick walk or a glass of water might fix the urge if hunger is not the cause.

### b. Keeping Sugary Treats Reasonable

- Occasional desserts can fit into a balanced lifestyle. Aim for moderate portions.

- If you have a sweet tooth, try fruit-based desserts or dark chocolate in small amounts.

- Do not let sweets become a daily habit that crowds out more nutritious foods.

---

## 5. Eating Out and Social Events

### a. Ordering Wisely

- Look for grilled, baked, or steamed options rather than fried.

- Choose sides like steamed veggies or a salad instead of fries if you want to keep the meal lighter.

- If servings are large, split the meal or take half home for another day.

### b. Balancing Party Foods

- At gatherings with lots of snacks, fill part of your plate with vegetables or fruit before sampling heavier dips or sweets.

- You do not have to avoid favorites; just keep an eye on portions to prevent overdoing it.

### c. Celebrating Without Guilt

- Special occasions are part of life. If you enjoy a richer meal, balance it out at the next meal by focusing on vegetables, lean protein, and water intake.

---

## 6. Personalizing for Ages and Stages

Remember the specific tips for children, teens, adults, and older adults:

- **Children:** Offer a variety of nutrient-rich foods in smaller, frequent meals. Model healthy habits.

- **Teens:** Support growth with enough protein, iron, and calcium. Encourage balanced choices even during busy schedules.

- **Young/Midlife Adults:** Plan around jobs or studies. Keep stress eating in check with prepared options.

- **Older Adults:** Focus on nutrient density, protein for muscle, and fiber plus hydration to support digestion.

---

## 7. Maintaining Heart Health and Steady Energy

### a. Heart-Supportive Choices

- Use unsaturated fats (like olive oil), lean proteins, and many fruits and vegetables.

- Limit overly salty, sugary, or highly processed foods.

- Keep an eye on portion sizes if weight management is a concern for blood pressure and cholesterol.

### b. Avoiding Energy Crashes

- Balanced meals with protein, complex carbs, and a little fat help keep you going without big highs or lows.

- Skipping meals or choosing only sugary snacks can cause sudden drops in blood sugar, leaving you drained.

---

## 8. Mindful Eating and Self-Care

### a. Listening to Hunger and Fullness

- Eat slowly, and notice when you start feeling satisfied. This helps you avoid overeating.

- Distracted eating, like scrolling on a phone or watching TV, can lead to missing your body's signals.

### b. Handling Emotions

- Stress, boredom, or sadness can push you to snack mindlessly. Identify the feeling before eating. If you are not truly hungry, try another form of relief (like a short break, gentle stretching, or a chat with a friend).

### c. Joy in Meals

- Cooking and eating can be enjoyable. Experiment with flavors, seasonings, and recipes. Share meals with family or friends for social support.

---

## 9. Overcoming Common Barriers

1. **Time Constraints**
   - Use batch cooking, simple recipes, or partial prep of ingredients (washing, chopping) to save time.
   - Consider cooking bigger portions that can feed you twice.

2. **Budget Concerns**
   - Focus on staple items: beans, lentils, oats, eggs (if you eat them), and seasonal produce.
   - Frozen vegetables are often cheaper and just as nutritious as fresh, particularly out of season.

3. **Picky Eating**
   - Offer a small portion of new foods alongside favorites. Give it time. People's tastes can change, and repeated gentle exposure helps.

4. **Limited Kitchen Skills**

    - Start with easy recipes (like scrambled eggs or a basic stir-fry). Gradually learn more.

    - Watch cooking videos or ask someone with experience to guide you.

---

## 10. Staying Motivated for the Long Run

### a. Setting Short-Term Goals

- "Add one extra serving of vegetables each day" or "Drink water instead of soda every other day" are small steps that feel doable.

- Once you master a goal, pick another.

### b. Tracking Progress

- Notice if you have more energy, improved sleep, or better mood. These changes can happen before bigger shifts in weight or body shape.

- Celebrating non-scale victories (like lifting heavier objects easily or feeling less stressed) boosts confidence.

### c. Building Routines

- Eating well becomes simpler when you have some habits. For example, deciding to have oatmeal or eggs for breakfast daily, or scheduling a grocery run every Saturday.

### d. Learning from Mistakes

- If you slip up for a day or week, do not give up. Reflect on what made it tough (lack of planning, stress, traveling) and plan around it next time.

---

## 11. A Sample Balanced Day

Below is an example to see how you might fit everything in. Adjust times and portion sizes to match your needs.

1. **Breakfast (7:00 AM)**

    - Oatmeal with milk (dairy or fortified plant-based), topped with sliced banana and a sprinkle of nuts.
    - Water or unsweetened tea.

2. **Mid-Morning Snack (10:00 AM)**

    - Carrot sticks with hummus or a small piece of fruit if hungry.

3. **Lunch (12:30 PM)**

    - Salad with leafy greens, chopped veggies, lean protein (chicken, tofu, or beans), and a whole-grain side (like a small piece of whole-grain bread).
    - Water to drink.

4. **Afternoon Pick-Me-Up (3:00 PM)**

    - Greek yogurt with berries or a handful of nuts.
    - Stay hydrated, sipping water or herbal tea.

5. **Dinner (6:30 PM)**

    - Baked fish or chicken, brown rice, and steamed or roasted vegetables (broccoli, carrots).
    - Season with herbs, garlic, or lemon juice instead of lots of salt.

6. **Optional Evening Snack (8:30 PM)**

    - If needed, a small mug of warm low-fat milk or a piece of fruit.
    - Avoid heavy, greasy foods before bed to support better sleep.

This pattern offers protein, complex carbs, vegetables, fruits, and hydration across the day. Portion sizes vary based on age, activity, and personal goals.

---

## 12. Building a Supportive Environment

### a. Family and Friends

- Involve them in meal planning, grocery shopping, or cooking. Having a "health buddy" can keep you accountable and inspired.

- Share recipes or do potluck dinners where each person contributes a nutritious dish.

**b. Workplace or School**

- Suggest or join a lunchtime walking group.

- If there are too many vending machine temptations, keep your own nutritious snacks in a drawer or cooler bag.

**c. Online and Community Resources**

- Many apps, websites, or local community centers offer tips, short videos, and meal ideas. Some have classes on basic cooking or healthy living.

- Be mindful of misinformation. Check credible sources like registered dietitians, reputable health organizations, or well-reviewed cookbooks.

---

## 13. Knowing When to Seek Professional Help

Sometimes, personalized advice is needed:

**1. Medical Conditions**

- If you have conditions like diabetes, heart concerns, or digestive issues, ask a doctor or dietitian how to adapt these guidelines safely.

- Certain medications might need special attention to diet.

### 2. Food Allergies or Intolerances

- If you suspect an allergy, consult a health professional for testing. Eliminating entire food groups without guidance can lead to nutrient gaps.

### 3. Ongoing Struggles

- If emotional eating, binge patterns, or very restrictive eating are happening, a counselor or specialist in eating behaviors can help.

---

## 14. Celebrating Your Progress

### a. Recognize Milestones

- Maybe you tried a new vegetable each week for a month or replaced daily soda with water. Recognize these achievements!

- Positive reinforcement can keep you eager for the next challenge.

### b. Reward Yourself (Non-Food Ways)

- Buy a new workout accessory, a comfortable pair of shoes, or a fun puzzle.

- Plan a day trip or do something enjoyable that aligns with your well-being.

### c. Pass On What You Learn

- Share cooking tips with friends or family. Encourage them if they want to make healthier choices. Teaching can reinforce your own knowledge.

## 15. A Lifelong Journey

Balanced eating is not a quick fix, but an ongoing journey. There might be phases in life—vacations, job changes, family expansions—where your routine shifts. By returning to the principles of variety, moderation, and balance, you can adapt without losing your progress. Your body thanks you when it gets the nutrients it needs, stays well-hydrated, and remains active. Over time, these daily decisions shape stronger habits and a healthier, more vibrant you.

## Conclusion of Chapter 20

You have now walked through each chapter of this fitness nutrition book, discovering how food and healthy habits can sustain a strong, energetic, and fulfilling life. From understanding the basics of proteins, carbs, and fats, to mastering meal planning, to guiding children, teens, and older adults, all these topics fit together like puzzle pieces. Here are the core reminders as you keep moving forward:

1. **Embrace Whole Foods:** Fruits, vegetables, whole grains, lean proteins, and healthy fats form the backbone of balanced meals.

2. **Plan Ahead:** Even small steps like writing a shopping list or batch-cooking a pot of rice make a big difference when time is tight.

3. **Stay Mindful:** Notice your hunger and fullness signals, manage stress without always turning to snacks, and savor your food.

4. **Balance Activity and Rest:** Physical movement pairs with proper rest and good nutrition to keep your body and mind at their best.

5. **Be Flexible:** There will be days when life feels hectic or celebrations pop up. Enjoy them, and return to your usual healthy habits afterward.

6. **Aim for Long-Term Consistency:** Change usually happens gradually, but small, steady actions can add up to remarkable benefits for your health, mood, and overall outlook.

By keeping these lessons in mind, you can face daily choices—be it at home, at a restaurant, or during a busy holiday season—armed with the knowledge to support your fitness and nutrition goals. This does not mean life will be without treats or quick fixes at times, but that you have the tools to maintain balance across the weeks and months. As you progress, remember to celebrate the improvements you notice, and keep exploring new foods, recipes, and activities that make healthy living both sustainable and enjoyable. Here's to a lifetime of feeling strong, nourished, and ready for whatever adventures come your way!

# Help Us Share Your Thoughts!

**Dear reader,**

Thank you for spending your time with this book. We hope it brought you enjoyment and a few new ideas to think about. If there was anything that didn't work for you, or if you have suggestions on how we can improve, please let us know at **kontakt@skriuwer.com**. Your feedback means a lot to us and helps us make our books even better.

If you enjoyed this book, we would be very grateful if you left a review on the site where you purchased it. Your review not only helps other readers find our books, but also encourages us to keep creating more stories and materials that you'll love.

By choosing Skriuwer, you're also supporting **Frisian**—a minority language mainly spoken in the northern Netherlands. Although **Frisian** has a rich history, the number of speakers is shrinking, and it's at risk of dying out. Your purchase helps fund resources to preserve and promote this language, such as educational programs and learning tools. If you'd like to learn more about Frisian or even start learning it yourself, please visit **www.learnfrisian.com**.

Thank you for being part of our community. We look forward to sharing more books with you in the future.

**Warm regards,**
The Skriuwer Team

www.ingramcontent.com/pod-product-compliance
Lightning Source LLC
LaVergne TN
LVHW012035070526
838202LV00056B/5510